THE LITTLE MONSTER

Growing Up with ADHD

Robert Jergen

ScarecrowEducation
Lanham, Maryland • Toronto • Oxford
2004

Published in the United States of America
by ScarecrowEducation
An imprint of The Rowman & Littlefield Publishing Group, Inc.
4501 Forbes Boulevard, Suite 200, Lanham, Maryland 20706
www.scarecroweducation.com

PO Box 317
Oxford
OX2 9RU, UK

British Library Cataloguing in Publication Information Available

Library of Congress Cataloging-in-Publication Data

Jergen, Robert.
    The little monster : growing up with ADHD / Robert Jergen.
        p. cm.
    ISBN 1-57886-104-7 (pbk.: alk. paper)
    1. Jergen, Robert. 2. Attention-deficit-disordered
children—Education—United States. 3. Attention-deficit-disordered
children—United States—Biography. 4. Attention-deficit hyperactivity
disorder. I. Title.
LC4713.4 .J47 2004
371.93—dc22

                                                        2003022783

⊗™ The paper used in this publication meets the minimum requirements of
American National Standard for Information Sciences—Permanence of Paper
for Printed Library Materials, ANSI/NISO Z39.48-1992.
Manufactured in the United States of America.

I would like to dedicate this book to the following life-forms:

Frank, my mentor, doctoral advisor, and friend. Frank was one of the few teachers in my life who actually enabled me to learn. I wouldn't be where I am today without Frank's help, encouragement, and support.

Nixon, Dante, Truman, Becky, Scout, all of the animals at the Humane Society, and especially the late Agnew. They always listen to me and treat me with love and respect.

And finally, Daisey, my love, partner, best friend, and everything else. She makes life worth living. I love you very, very much, Peanut.

CONTENTS

Acknowledgments   vii

Preface   ix

A Brief Overview of ADHD—Understanding the Power   xiii

1 Meet the Jergens   1

2 Welcome to My World   5

3 Send in the Teachers   23

4 Junior High: Heroes and Hope Gone   35

5 Hobbits, High School, and New Homes   45

6 Boilermakers and Fuzzy Navels   59

7 Rebecca and the Adult World   73

8 EEG, MRI, A-OK   81

9 Storming the Gates of the Ivory Tower   97

10 Life after School   105

11 A Look at the Present   119

12 Strategies for Changing My Environments   123

13 Strategies for Learning to Learn   135

14 Strategies for Building Emotional Support   145

15 A Look Behind   155

16 A Look Forward   165

17 Some Suggestions for Parents, Teachers, and People
        with ADHD   171

About the Author   179

ACKNOWLEDGMENTS

Before we begin, I would like to acknowledge the many people without whom this book probably would not be necessary or published.

First, I want to acknowledge Tom Koerner, the vice president of ScarecrowEducation. Tom is not only a wonderful person but also a fantastic editor. He encouraged me to send him proposal after proposal and returned all of my numerous e-mails with astonishing punctuality. You probably wouldn't be reading this book if it had not been for Tom and all of the terrific people at Scarecrow.

I also want to acknowledge my agent, Bert Krages. Bert worked very hard approaching publishers and negotiating contracts for this project.

Finally, I want to acknowledge my parents, family, friends, and all of the teachers, counselors, and doctors who have been involved in my life. As you will see, I have not always liked what they said or did to me, but I realize that they have helped make me who I am today. So please, blame them.

PREFACE

When I mentioned to my friends and family that I planned on writing an autobiography, nearly all of them looked at me slightly puzzled and asked why. After all, as some of them asked, "Who would want to read about *your* life?"

It is a fair question. I haven't cured cancer, spied for a foreign country, or killed anybody. I am not a rock or movie star. I haven't played professional sports or made a billion dollars on the stock market. In fact, I haven't done anything infamous or terribly spectacular in any way. Still, I think that what I have done will be of some interest to a great many people, especially parents, teachers, and more than 8.5 million children in the United States alone.

You see, in 1993, at the age of twenty-four, I was diagnosed with ADHD. At that very moment, a lifetime of pain, rejection, and failure was suddenly explained to me. I went from thinking that I was a freak and that I would eventually go completely crazy to realizing that I was just different and that was okay. I also realized that I wasn't alone.

I spent the remainder of my twenties trying to find ways of making ADHD an asset. I literally sat down and developed strategies and accommodations that made ADHD a "super ability." I learned how to construct an environment in which I could be productive. I learned how to teach myself what I needed to know. And, most important, I learned how to deal with the emotional baggage that comes from years of disappointment and failure.

As a result, I have become pretty "successful" in my life. Specifically, by age thirty-four, I have earned a Ph.D. in special education in half the time as my non-ADHD peers. I became an associate professor and published more in a few years than many academics publish throughout their entire lives. I have won awards, written reports to Congress, been interviewed by *Time* magazine, and presented all over the country. I have my own house, a beautiful girlfriend who loves and respects me, and—I have to say, I have a wonderful life.

With this book, I am not offering any pat answers. The road to Nirvana is an individualized one and I am afraid that I can't truly help anybody but myself. Nonetheless, through this book, I will attempt to accomplish three things.

The first is to explain to "normal" people what it is like having ADHD. Parents, teachers, social workers, counselors, and the myriad of other professionals who work with children with ADHD cannot help these kids without first appreciating what their lives are like. Unfortunately, after reading everything that I could get my hands on, I realized that there are currently no books that accurately discuss ADHD from the perspective of the child. Additionally, the literature that is out there makes ADHD sound as if it is some sort of horrible infliction from the Middle Ages—which, as you will soon see, is simply not true.

Second, I outline some of the strategies that have helped me find happiness and success. I go through the process that I used to develop these approaches as well as my rationale behind them. Perhaps, through this exploration, you will find something that works for you or your child.

Finally, it is my greatest desire that, through investigating the good and bad of my life, I can give people hope. In and of itself, ADHD is not a bad thing. As I will say over and over again, it is a powerful gift—if it is utilized properly. I have ADHD. I am glad that I have ADHD. I wouldn't want to be any other way. I will even go so far as to say that, if I ever have children, I hope that they will have ADHD, too. In short, having ADHD is A-OK! By the time you get to the end of this book, I am betting that you will agree.

Before you begin reading, I need to point out that I have tried to be as accurate as possible in retelling these stories. I have relied upon a wealth of notes from my former teachers as well as observations provided by my friends, family, and coworkers. Whenever possible, I have tried to quote people as best as I am able. But, as we will discuss, people with ADHD have faulty memories. Moreover, many of these events happened while I was very young or drinking. Still, I believe that I have given some resemblance of the "truth," although others in my life might disagree.

I also want to point out that I tell a lot of stories involving my family. I give particular emphasis to how they responded to my "uniqueness." As a result, they might come across as ogres. They aren't. They were, and are, good people. I just frustrated them and they didn't know how to deal with me. Still, I believe that people can learn from these stories and find some sort of comfort in the notion that somebody like me turned out more or less okay.

A BRIEF OVERVIEW OF ADHD— UNDERSTANDING THE POWER

ADHD (attention deficit hyperactivity disorder) is a neurological condition characterized by difficulty regulating activity, impulses, and attention. It is thought to be caused by an irregularity in the brain. Specifically, research has suggested that people with ADHD have "abnormal" brainstems and frontal lobes that control behavior and attention, respectively.

Over the past decade or so, ADHD has become extremely common. It seems that you cannot read a newspaper or watch a television program without coming across some reference to it. In fact, recent studies have indicated that roughly 5 to 7 percent of children in the United States have some form of ADHD. That is approximately 8.5 million children in the United States alone! When adults are included, this number is likely to more than double.

However, back when I was born in the late 1960s, ADHD didn't exist. That is to say, the term was not yet used (see table 1). Children who displayed symptoms of ADHD thirty years ago might have been diagnosed with "minimal brain dysfunction" (MBD). The idea was that the brains of these children were damaged, possibly by the use of forceps during delivery. This slight injury to the brain caused children to run around uncontrollably, act impulsively, and have difficulty paying attention—or at least, that was the theory.

Table I.   A Brief History of ADHD

1900	Dr. George Still describes children with poor impulse and motor control.
1950s	Minimal brain dysfunction (MBD) becomes a diagnosable condition for children who have problems maintaining attention.
1970s	Hyperkinetic reaction disorder (HRD) because a diagnosable condition for children who have problems controlling their activity level.
1980s	The terms "attention deficit hyperactivity disorder" (ADHD) and "attention deficit disorder" (ADD) are first coined.
1990s	The American Psychiatric Association drops the use of ADD as a viable diagnosis and separates ADHD into four subtypes: ADHD–Inattentive Type (ADHD-I), ADHD–Hyperactive-Impulsive Type (ADHD-HI), ADHD–Combined Type (ADHD-C), and ADHD–Not Otherwise Specified (ADHD-NOS).

Even though minimal brain dysfunction was a legitimate medical condition, few children at the time were diagnosed with it. This probably wasn't due to its actual prevalence being low. More likely, the lack of diagnosis was because few doctors and teachers had heard of, or were looking for, it. After all, pre-1975 special education was mainly reserved for children with severe and multiple disabilities, or perhaps "obvious" disabilities such as Down syndrome or blindness. Consequently, students who had minimal brain dysfunction were not routinely identified.

Back in the early 1970s, children with minimal brain dysfunction were not considered "disabled" in the way children with ADHD are today, nor were they given specialized programs or medications. They were simply "problem" students who were frequently kicked out of class and sent to the principal's office. Further, the only behavior modification that children with minimal brain dysfunction received came predominantly in the form of good old-fashioned spankings.

In 1975, a law called the Education for All Handicapped Children Act (EAHCA), also known as P.L. 94-142, was enacted. It mandated that all children with disabilities from age six to twenty-one were to be provided a free and appropriate public education in the least restrictive environment possible. P.L. 94-142 also directs that schools actively attempt to identify students who have disabilities that adversely affect their ability to learn. As a result of this overt search, the number of kids identified with disabilities skyrocketed.

By the mid-1980s, the public was becoming more and more aware of a wide array of disabilities, such as dyslexia, fetal alcohol syndrome, and behavior disorders. Advocacy groups for people with disabilities and their parents were springing up in nearly every community. The popular media portrayed people with disabilities on such television programs as *Life Goes On* and *The Facts of Life*, and teachers became better skilled at diagnosing previously underidentified conditions. Consequently, students with disabilities were being recognized and placed in special education at even higher rates than during the beginning of the decade.

Also by the mid-1980s, the term "minimal brain dysfunction" was discontinued as a medical diagnosis. Individuals with symptoms related to minimal brain dysfunction were now considered to have either "attention deficit disorder" (ADD) or "attention deficit hyperactivity disorder" (ADHD).

ADD was characterized by the inability to pay attention. Students with ADD would stare out the window, make careless mistakes, and miss important details. They would also have difficulty following conversations and making coherent arguments that followed a logical train of thought.

ADHD was characterized by the inability to regulate motor activity. Students with ADHD would likely fidget in their chairs, move around excessively, talk fast, have difficulty waiting their turns, and rush through their homework. They would also have problems being impulsive, such as saying or doing things without thinking.

In the early 1990s, several studies began to find that many children had problems with attention as well as with hyperactivity. According to diagnosis procedures, however, these children could not have both ADD and ADHD. They had to have one or the other. Questions arose regarding what to do with students who qualified for both conditions.

Because of this confusion, the American Psychiatric Association (APA) rewrote the criteria used to diagnose students with ADD and ADHD. Specifically, they dropped the term "attention deficit disorder." So, despite what is reported in the media, ADD is no longer a recognized diagnosis. Moreover, they made attention deficit hyperactivity disorder an umbrella term that includes four specific conditions.

The first condition is attention deficit hyperactivity disorder, predominantly inattentive type (or ADHD-I). According to the latest edition of APA's *Diagnostic and Statistical Manual of Mental Disorders* (DSM),[1]

ADHD-I is characterized by six or more of the following symptoms over a six-month period:

- Often fails to give close attention to details or makes careless mistakes in schoolwork, work, or other activities
- Often has difficulty sustaining attention in tasks or play activities
- Often does not seem to listen when spoken to directly
- Often does not follow though on instructions and fails to finish schoolwork, chores, or duties in the workplace (not due to oppositional behavior or failure to understand instructions)
- Often has difficulty organizing tasks and activities
- Often avoids, dislikes, or is reluctant to engage in tasks that require sustained mental effort (such as schoolwork or homework)
- Often loses things necessary for tasks or activities (e.g., toys, school assignments, pencils, books, or tools)
- Is often easily distracted by extraneous stimuli
- Is often forgetful in daily activities[2]

ADHD-I is very similar to the ADD of the 1980s. However, whereas individuals need to exhibit a minimum of six symptoms in order to have ADHD-I, at least eight symptoms were needed for ADD. In other words, it is easier to have ADHD-I now than it was to have ADD twenty years ago. This could explain why ADHD is becoming more and more widespread.

The second condition identified by APA in the 1990s is attention deficit hyperactivity disorder, predominantly hyperactive-impulsive type (or ADHD-HI). ADHD-HI is very similar to the ADHD of the 1980s. But, as with ADD and ADHD-I, fewer symptoms are needed to have ADHD-HI than ADHD. According to the fourth revised edition of *DSM*, individuals need to display at least six of the following symptoms over a minimum of six consecutive months:

- Often fidgets with hands or feet or squirms in seat
- Often leaves seat in classroom or in other situations in which remaining seated is expected
- Often runs about or climbs excessively in situations in which it is inappropriate (in adolescents or adults, may be limited to subjective feelings of restlessness)

- Often has difficulty playing or engaging in leisure activities quietly
- Is often "on the go" or often acts as if "driven by a motor"
- Often talks excessively
- Often blurts out answers before questions have been completed
- Often has difficulty awaiting turn
- Often interrupts or intrudes on others (e.g., butts into conversations or games)

In addition to the criteria listed above, people with ADHD-I and ADHD-HI must also fulfill three other criteria. Specifically, they must display some of their symptoms prior to age seven. So an adolescent who suddenly has trouble paying attention or sitting quietly would not have any form of ADHD. He or she could just be going through the normal changes that occur during their passage to adulthood or perhaps he or she is beginning to abuse drugs.

Additionally, in order to have ADHD, the symptoms must be inconsistent with the person's developmental age. This means that their behaviors have to be compared to those of their peers. Clearly, all three-year-olds are likely to say things without thinking or become restless when bored. This doesn't mean that they have ADHD. It is simply how they are supposed to behave.

Not only do the behaviors of individuals with ADHD have to be different from their peers, they also have to produce a significant impairment to the person's functioning ability in multiple environments. In other words, in order to have ADHD, a person's inattentiveness or hyperactivity has to create such a problem that he has trouble learning or working or socializing. Additionally, the difficulties must exist in more than one location. So if a child has all of the symptoms listed earlier, but only in her science class, she would not have ADHD. She probably is just bored or tired or in love with the person next to her or any one of the near infinite number of other potential explanations.

Finally, according to APA's diagnostic procedures, the symptoms of ADHD cannot be caused by some other condition or situation. For example, individuals who are hyperactive or impulsive because they take amphetamines would not have any form of ADHD. The same is true if somebody didn't pay attention because he had a hearing impairment or was depressed because he had a death in the family.

This is not to say that people with ADHD cannot have multiple disabilities. We can. In fact, as many as 70 percent of children with ADHD also have other diagnoses, such as obsessive-compulsive disorder (OCD), Tourette's syndrome, dyslexia, and anxiety disorders. However, the symptoms of ADHD cannot be caused by these other conditions.

To address the issue of what to do when somebody meets the criteria for both ADHD-I and ADHD-HI, APA developed ADHD-C, or attention deficit hyperactivity disorder, combined type. These individuals are not only inattentive but also hyperactive and impulsive. As you will learn later, this is the type of ADHD that I have.

The final category of ADHD is called ADHD-NOS, or "not otherwise specified." This is often referred to as "pseudo-ADHD." While individuals with ADHD-I and ADHD-HI need to exhibit at least six symptoms, people with ADHD-NOS do not need to have as many. In other words, ADHD-NOS is for people who clearly have problems with hyperactivity, impulsivity, or inattention to such a degree that their lives are adversely affected, but they do not have enough symptoms to be classified as having any other ADHD. In effect, you might think of it as a "milder" form of ADHD.

Of the three main forms of ADHD (e.g., ADHD-I, -HI, and -C), approximately 55 percent of people have ADHD-C, while 27 percent have ADHD-I and the remaining 18 percent have ADHD-HI. Further, boys are seven times more likely to be diagnosed with an ADHD than are girls. When girls have ADHD, they are more likely to have ADHD-I than any other type.

Since the mid-1990s, the number of children who have been identified with attention disorders has mushroomed by over 300 percent. The reason for this huge increase is hotly debated. Yes, as I mentioned, the criteria used to diagnose these disorders has changed significantly over the past couple of decades, making it easier to have some form of ADHD. And, yes, people are more aware of ADHD than ever before, so individuals are referred for evaluations more often than in previous years. Still, these factors probably only account for part of the increase. A more plausible explanation is likely to lie with pharmaceutical companies.

Before the mid-1990s, approximately 6 percent of children who had ADHD were treated with medication. By the end of the decade, this number increased to more than 80 percent. In fact, in 2002, more than two million children in the United States were on Ritalin. When other medications are included, it is likely that two or three students in every classroom in America are on some sort of drug for ADHD.

The principal reason for the incredible proliferation of ADHD, and the use of pharmaceuticals to treat it, is probably more economic than medical in nature. Where there is money to be made, companies will create a demand for their products. If they could, they would convince every parent that his or her kid has ADHD and should be on their product.

Don't get me wrong. This isn't a knock against the pharmaceutical companies. After all, this is what businesses are supposed to do. They are supposed to make money, not to teach children. It would be unfair to expect them to do otherwise.

The responsibility for the escalation of ADHD lies predominantly with teachers and parents. ADHD has become very fashionable. It is much easier for parents and teachers to claim that their children have ADHD than a less palatable diagnosis of "behavior disorder." Specifically, a diagnosis of ADHD is more advantageous than behavior disorder in two ways.

First, according to the media, ADHD can be "cured" quickly and easily by pills. There are few such remedies for other conditions. For instance, when a child has oppositional defiant disorder (ODD), she is usually "treated" using systematic behavior modification programs that reinforce appropriate behavior. These programs take more time and effort than giving medications.

Second, diagnosing a child with ADHD minimizes the shame that many parents and teachers experience when they have an unruly kid. With the diagnosis of ADHD, parents and teachers can say, "It isn't my fault. They have a malfunctioning brain."

Because of this, many people claim that ADHD is overdiagnosed. Maybe it is. Clearly, people are mislabeled with ADHD. But many people have ADHD and don't realize it. Still, the biggest issue is not whether there should be more or fewer people with attention problems. The biggest issue is the public's misconception of what ADHD is.

Watch television or listen to people talk. The general consensus is that ADHD is some sort of horrible, debilitating disability that has to be eradicated from the face of the earth. This is unfortunate given that there are many positive aspects to having ADHD. For example, people with ADHD tend to be very smart or even cognitively gifted. They can also be very creative and funny, such as Robin Williams and Jim Carrey—both of whom have ADHD. Further, as covered throughout this book, people with ADHD can become extremely productive and successful. However, without appreciating the true nature of ADHD, people will not fully utilize these natural abilities.

Think about it this way. Who wouldn't want to have more energy? Who wouldn't want to be creative or think differently than everybody else? These are the natural characteristics of people with ADHD. So ADHD is a gift, not a disability! Perhaps, in the future, all parents will hope that their kids will have ADHD. Perhaps, in the future, everybody will be glad that they have ADHD. I know that I do.

NOTES

1. At the time of this book's writing, the latest version of the *Diagnostic and Statistical Manual of Mental Disorders* (DSM) was the revised fourth edition or DSM-IV-TR. The DSM is updated every few years. For the most accurate information, make sure that you have the most recent publication.

2. American Psychiatric Association. *Diagnostic and Statistical Manual of Mental Disorders*, 4th ed. Washington, D.C.: APA, 2000.

1

MEET THE JERGENS

I am the youngest of five boys.

My oldest brother, Jim, is the smart one. He is a neurologist, or, as my mother says, the "real" doctor of the family. He always did well in school and, as far as I know, never got a grade below an A. When I had Jim's former teachers, they always expected me to be as intelligent as he was. After grading my assignments, they quickly became disillusioned. I was inconsistent, made ridiculous mistakes, and had great difficulty focusing on even the simplest tasks.

Glenn is the second oldest. He was the superstar athlete of the family. He wrestled, ran track, and played football and baseball. In college, he scored four touchdowns in one game! When I was about to enter high school, the football, baseball, and wrestling coaches all tried to convince me to join their teams. When they watched me play, they weren't very impressed. Although I was very active, I was uncoordinated and highly distractible. During a baseball game, a pop fly bounced off my head when I wasn't looking. This happened twice—in the same game!

John is the middle child. He is the sweet one, the big teddy bear of the family. Once he was wrestling and his opponent started screaming in pain. John let him go because he didn't want to hurt anybody. That is just how he was. Everybody liked John. People didn't like me. I said things that people thought were rude or arrogant or obnoxious. I didn't mean to; asinine things just popped out of my mouth without me realizing it. As a result, I didn't have many friends when I was growing up. I still don't.

Richard is the second youngest. He is the funny one, the comedian of the family. He performs at the local comedy clubs, often telling jokes about me. He is always good for a laugh. When I meet people who know Rich, they expect me to zing off good one-liners or say something clever. I try, but I usually say something completely inappropriate or incoherent and they walk away muttering to themselves.

Then there is me—Robert, or Robbie as most of my family calls me. I am the strange one. The melodramatic, emotional one. The one whom everybody looked at when something was broken or missing. The one at whom they would roll their eyes and shake their heads. I am the freak, the loser, the "overly sensitive" one, the slob, the underachiever, the social oddity. I was, and am, as foreign to my family as a chocolate-flavored hot dog.

My mother is first-generation American. Her mother was from Stavanger, Norway. My maternal grandfather was from Stockholm, Sweden. So my mother grew up with a strong sense of family and priority to education that is typical in Scandinavian countries. Further, she did not believe in spanking, which is also typical for Scandinavians. My father, on the other hand, was from a completely different background.

My father's family is Bohemian by origin. I am not sure when they came to the United States, but it must have been several generations ago. So long ago, in fact, that they still identify themselves as Bohemians and not Czech. He brought to our family an extremely strong work ethic and a sense of discipline. He, unlike my mother, *did* believe in spanking and I frequently found myself bent over his knees.

I think that my antics frustrated my father far more than they did my mother. He was not a very tolerant man and he expected his children to be in control of themselves at all times. My mother was more patient and logical, but she could not see any logic in my behavior, which confused her endlessly. Clearly, I tried both of their patience on a nearly daily basis.

How a Norwegian-Swede from Brooklyn, New York, married a Bohemian from the suburbs of Chicago is a very long story that is probably only interesting to my immediate family. Suffice it to say that they met during the Korean War while my father was stationed with the Navy in Manhattan. They danced at a YMCA social and, after several rejections, my mother finally agreed to marry my father. They eventually moved to Beach Grove, Illinois, and had five strapping baby boys. This is where I come in.

2

WELCOME TO MY WORLD

Beach Grove, Illinois, is a suburban town twenty-five miles due west of Chicago. When I was growing up during the 1970s, it had approximately 40,000 people and was overwhelmingly white and middle class. There was little crime. The schools were good. We played in the streets, knew our neighbors, and felt safe. The biggest scandals involved the people living behind us throwing a loud party past 10 o'clock or somebody letting their lawn grow too high.

In short, Beach Grove was much like the setting for a 1950s family television show and, although our house didn't have a white picket fence or a tire swing, our family certainly played its part. We were like the Cleavers on *Leave It to Beaver* or the Cunninghams on *Happy Days*.

We ate dinners together. We belonged to a country club where we swam during the hot Illinois summers. During the Easter and Christmas holidays, my mother dressed us in matching outfits, sometimes with little bow ties, and we visited our grandparents in the next town nearly every weekend. When our dog Frisky had puppies, we even held a family meeting to decide which of them we were going to keep. We were the clean-cut, all-American, suburban family living the American dream.

Most people in Beach Grove knew us one way or another. My mother was president of the PTA for a while. My father coached a couple of Little

League baseball teams. My paternal grandfather was known as Uncle Louie and had a park named after him. Plus, my brothers were all very noteworthy in their respective areas. As I said before, Jim was very smart, Glenn was the wrestling champion for the local high school, John was big and cuddly, and Richard was funny. All we needed was a theme song and we could have been the Brady Bunch or the Partridge Family.

I was born at Hillside Hospital on September 14, 1968. As far as I know, there was no terrible storm with lightning flashing every time my mother had a contraction. There was no eclipse of the sun or moon. Nor were there locusts swarming over the town.

I am told that the pregnancy, although "unplanned," was without any complications. My mother never smoked or drank or failed to gain an appropriate amount of weight. Further, I went full term and she had all of the prenatal care that was expected at that time.

I am also told that the delivery was unremarkable. I was not a blue baby or had any physical ailments except for slightly pigeon-toed feet, which were quickly corrected by casts. Moreover, despite what my brothers would later tell me, I didn't have a twin that they sold into slavery and the doctor didn't drop me on my head. From all appearances, I was a perfectly normal eight-pound, ten-ounce baby boy.

The fact that I am part of a fairly large family, as well as the youngest, is an important point to keep in mind. You see, in special education, there is a term called "parental frame of reference." Basically, parents who only have one child usually do not have much of a basis for comparison. Consequently, they tend to either see things wrong with children who are completely normal or they see their special needs children as perfect in every way. Having had four other boys before they had me, my parents knew exactly what to expect. So, even as an infant, they knew that I was different.

As my mother tells it, as soon as my big brown eyes popped open after a nap, my arms and legs would be moving around so frantically that the crib would tremble. From the very beginning, I was raring to go. As soon as I was able to crawl, which was at five months thank you very much, I was racing around the house and getting into trouble. I wouldn't sit still or sleep for very long. I broke everything that I could get my hands on and I was constantly making noise, as my father would say, "just for the sake of making noise." I was so active that my mother used to call me her "little monster"—a name that stuck.

In all fairness, I wasn't the best of kids, as you will soon find out. My parents had a difficult time raising me. As patient as my mother could be, she would frequently clench her fists and her jaw, look heavenward, and say, "Jesus Christ, give me strength! You are such a rotten kid!" My father would shake his head and roll his eyes when he looked at me. His brow furrowed in a kind of roadmap to frustration.

It should be noted that my mother denies ever saying, "Jesus Christ, give me strength! You are such a rotten kid!" She says that she said a simple prayer every time I tested her patience—something like, "Lord, give me strength to deal with these trying times." Nevertheless, our long-term neighbors and honorary members of our family, the Scholzes, have confirmed that my mother did, in fact, say that I was a rotten kid. The frequency of these comments is still being vehemently debated.

This raises another very important point to consider. Whether my mother and father showed their disapproval of me and my behavior every minute of every day, or whether it was simply once as a passing comment, doesn't really matter. You see, people with ADHD have a very poor perception of reality. This is not to say that we are crazy, although for many years I thought that I was. It is just that we tend to obsess on things. For example, you might have had a song running uncontrollably through your head for hours at a time. I have had my mother saying, "Jesus Christ, give me strength! You are such a rotten kid!" echoing in my mind for over thirty years. It is how I will always picture my mother, looking upward so angry that she could barely control herself, telling me that I was a rotten kid. I suspect that when she is dead, I will still hear her saying this over and over. So it is not completely clear to me whether my mother actually said what she said over and over or whether I am just replaying a memory of one specific event. Either way, my reality was that I was a rotten kid and sometimes I misbehaved purely to play the part.

In special education, we call this a "self-fulfilling prophecy." Kids become what they are told that they are. Had my family and teachers told me that I was wonderful and smart and caring, most of my odd behaviors probably would have gone away or at least been less bizarre. Instead, they focused almost exclusively on what I did wrong. So, consequently, what I did wrong became largely who I was. I was, and in my mind still am, a screwup.

Please note that I am not blaming my parents. They are fabulous people who tried their best to care for and provide me with everything that
I needed. I never went without anything. I was never abused. I was
never neglected. They loved me and did what they could to give me a
good life. They raised me like they raised their other four, non-ADHD
sons. Perhaps that was the problem.

I wasn't like my brothers, as my mother still points out. I was extremely
active and always talking or doing something. If I wasn't building things,
I was destroying them. Or I was running around, climbing over the fur-
niture, jumping down the stairs, swinging from tree branches, or a hundred and one other things all within moments of each other. I tried my
best to behave. I really did. I wanted to be a good kid, but I frequently
did things without thinking or without even realizing that I did them.

I also took everything to heart. I was hyperemotional and easily
crushed. While my mother's curses and my father's eye rolling didn't
seem to affect my brothers, they devastated me. When my parents
called me a rotten kid, or my brothers teased me, I would fall apart. I
would crumble as if the world was coming to an end and there was nothing left to live for. From the very beginning, I was ultra thin-skinned and
everybody had to walk on eggshells around me. Perhaps some stories
about the little monster would help give you a sense of what my parents
and brothers had to endure.

My brothers tell the story about me and my pacifier. Apparently, one
night when I was very young, my mother had gone out leaving my father
to watch the five Jergen children. Sometime during the night, I lost my
pacifier and I started screaming. I screamed and screamed and
screamed until my father got all of the brothers out of bed and conducted a systematic room-by-room search of the house. Nobody was allowed to sleep until my pacifier was found.

Okay, you are probably thinking, "Big deal. That happened when I
was a kid, too. Kids lose things and they drive their parents nuts until
they are found." Yes, this is true. But when I was a child, that kind of
thing happened with great regularity. I constantly lost things. Further, I
had a horrible time dealing with change and disappointment.

Like most kids with ADHD, I was *extremely* sensitive. Every little minor setback was a major catastrophe. When something went wrong, I
couldn't seem to get over it. I obsessed about things and couldn't let

them go. Even thoughts of imaginary problems produced massive amounts of anxiety that would diminish my capacity to function. I was a giant, raw, throbbing nerve that would flinch in pain with the slightest provocation, whether it was real or contrived.

This extreme reaction relates back to how our minds work. For instance, you might have a thought come into your head, it stays a little while, and then it leaves. Maybe you have even had a song or a jingle going through your head for a couple of days at a time. It is kind of annoying, isn't it?

Now add three or four or five more thoughts to the mix and amplify them. Spin them round and round and round in your head and make them go faster and faster and faster until they become like an all-consuming obsession. Everything centers on those thoughts. You can't focus on anything else. You can't escape them. They drive you insane. That is what it is like having ADHD.

When I got upset as a child, I would go from being completely fine to wailing like a banshee for hours. I couldn't control it. No matter how frequently I was spanked or punished, I simply could not control my emotions or my reactions to them. I felt, and still feel, things with such intensity that it is very hard for me to "unfeel" them or to get them out of my head. So, whenever I lost my pacifier or stuffed bunny rabbit, felt ignored, was picked on by my brothers, experienced any kind of injustice, or whatever, I had a meltdown of biblical proportions.

Keep in mind that I lost things *a lot*, which, as we talked about earlier, is a defining characteristic of ADHD. So my tantrums were not just a once-in-a-while occurrence. They happened nearly every day.

Further, these extremely strong attachments and feelings were something totally different from what my normal brothers displayed when they were my age. When they lost their pacifier, they might cry, but my mother could usually get them wanting something else. She could distract them and calm them down. When I lost my pacifier, I went ballistic. I went berserk! My parents simply could not understand what the fuss was about. The sheer intensity of my emotions scared them. My brothers never went through that stage and my parents were caught completely off guard.

This kind of behavior is very common for kids with ADHD. While we often appear oblivious to everything around us, we also become so single-minded that we think the world is falling apart when little things go wrong. We have addictive personalities that can't let go. Just like how my mind constantly replays my mother saying "Jesus Christ, give me strength! You are such a rotten kid," my mind also locks onto other things and will not let them go.

For instance, just last night, I couldn't fall asleep until I went and bought a sprinkler for my garden. It sounds stupid but at two in the morning on a work night, I had to get up out of bed, drive to the twenty-four-hour Wal-Mart to buy a stupid sprinkler. All I could think about was this damned sprinkler and how I needed one. Sprinkler! Sprinkler! Sprinkler! My mind was locked and I couldn't unlock it and go to sleep until I did its bidding.

My parents and teachers never understood that aspect of me. To be honest, for many years, I didn't either. I just thought that I was insane—literally, insane. But my fanatical single-mindedness wasn't the only behavior that I had that my normal brothers never displayed.

I was always on the go. I was always running or climbing or screaming or doing something that required constant supervision. My mother couldn't keep her eye on me and my four older brothers at the same time, so I frequently got into mischief when she wasn't looking.

For example, when I was two years old or so, I was able to figure out how to unlock and open the back door to the house. My mother attempted to block it so I couldn't escape, but I would be able to get out somehow. Further, I was able to unlatch the gate leading out of our backyard.

One day, wearing nothing but a diaper, I broke out of the Jergen prison and waddled through the backyard, down the alley, and down Main Street. My father saw me on a corner of one of the busiest intersections in town as he was coming home from work. Boy, was my mother surprised when he came home with me tucked under one arm! After a while, it happened with such regularity that she stopped being surprised at all. She was just grateful that I hadn't been hit by a car or abducted.

Her concerns were well founded. I had no sense of danger. I would throw knives, play with fire, touch hot burners on the stove, mix chemicals, and put things in electrical sockets. Once I ran out into the street and my grandmother had to grab my arm so that I didn't get run over. She actually dislocated my shoulder. Another time I cut my left index finger down to the bone as I fooled around with a razor blade. I still have the scar.

When I was three or four, I had heard my brothers talking about baseball cards and autographs. They used to go watch the Chicago White Sox or the Cubs play and would come back with autographs of famous players. Somehow I got it into my head that a person's name written on a piece of paper was worth a lot of money. I became fixated on this idea of names equaling money. I remember that I just couldn't let it go.

So, early one morning, I got up, scribbled on some pieces of paper (I didn't know how to write my name yet), and then went door-to-door trying to sell my autograph. It was probably about 5:00 in the morning, if not earlier. People were not happy to see the little monster banging on their door. I vaguely remember some elderly woman smiling down at me and offering me a cookie for the slip of paper with crayon markings on it. I also remember getting very upset and demanding a dollar before I stomped away with no cookie and no dollar.

I think that incident, or perhaps the many more that followed, caused some of the older neighbors on the block to look down upon my mother. Again, it was the late 1960s to early 1970s. Many people still thought that a woman's place was in the home and several of the older neighbors made sarcastic comments to my mother about doing a better job raising her kids—more precisely, raising me.

I still feel badly about that. My mother was a good mother despite what they thought. She had five boys within ten years. She couldn't be everywhere at once and we didn't have a housekeeper like the Brady Bunch.

My mother's experiences were pretty representative of most parents who have children with ADHD. Undertaking ordinary daily activities was very challenging for her. For example, going to the grocery store was a disaster waiting to happen. Every shelf or display was a potential play area for me. I would run around screaming, knocking things over, causing a mess wherever I went.

Our neighbor, Mrs. Scholz, tells a funny story about how she always knew whether my mother and I were in a store. Apparently, as soon as she entered the building, she would hear me screaming and then an announcement over the public address system would say, "Cleanup on aisle three!" Of course, she heard my mother screaming, too. Cries of "Rob, stop that!" "Put that down!" "Leave that alone!" "Rob, stop that! I mean it!" floated from aisle to aisle. Unfortunately, my behaviors were not confined to stores.

Every year, we would go to New York to see my mother's family. Once we took the train. According to my parents, I ran up and down the car singing "Twinkle, Twinkle, Little Star" nearly the entire way there. Several of the other passengers told my mother to "Shut that kid up!" But there was nothing she could do. She could distract me, but only for a second or two. She could try to get me to sleep, but that would only work if my energy was about to run out. I simply could not sit or play quietly. I had to be moving. I had to be making noise. I had to be exploring everything and everybody! We only took the train once.

After we stopped taking the train, we started driving. Having two adults, five children, and a dog in the fake-wood-paneled station wagon for sixteen hours made my father a chain-smoker. Every few minutes I would ask him, "How much longer?" or "Are we there yet?" I knew that I was being annoying. I tried to be quiet. But the questions kept popping out of my mouth. I couldn't stop them. Thankfully, I sat way in the back, well out of my father's reach.

Again, there is an extremely important issue to consider here. The child is not the only one affected by ADHD. We cause a great deal of stress and frustration for everybody around us and parents often feel that they are causing their child's poor behavior, or at the very least allowing it to continue. They also tend to feel as if they are "bad parents," which, of course, can create a profound sense of guilt and shame. These feeling are magnified by the numerous angry looks and stares that parents get when their children misbehave in public.

I have heard many stories from parents of children with ADHD on this topic and they are almost always heart-wrenching. For instance, I know several couples who are no longer speaking to their own parents because the grandparents feel the grandchild with ADHD is "out of control." The grandparents say that the parents are "too lenient" and need to discipline their kids more often.

I also know of many grandparents who refuse to baby-sit their grandchildren—some because they physically cannot keep up with the child with ADHD, and others who simply can't tolerate the child's obnoxious behavior.

Moreover, I have witnessed teachers yelling at parents for not putting their children on drugs. Once, I was at an individualized education program (IEP) meeting where a teacher actually accused the parents of "abusing" their child because they refused to put the student on Ritalin! Abuse! Can you believe it? The teacher actually implied that she was going to get child protective services involved!

Clearly, all parents sacrifice part of their spousal relationship to some degree when they have children. When a baby is born, much of the time has to be dedicated to its care. As a result, the parents can't be a couple as much as they used to be. This is just natural.

But imagine what it is like when the child has ADHD. Imagine having to give him or her constant attention and supervision. The child runs around, gets into everything, and never gives the parents a moment's peace. Imagine trying to get the child to behave, but nothing works. Inevitably, stress is going to build and, if it is not released properly, parents usually either start to fight or shut down. Understandably, there is a high divorce rate among parents of special needs children, including those with ADHD.

In all fairness, ADHD affects teachers just as much as parents, although admittedly in different ways. Teachers only have to deal with these children for a few hours a day, five days a week. They also have the luxury of blaming parents for their child's poor behavior. Parents spend far more time with the children and do not have summers off. Further, they have to live with a lifetime of guilt and what-ifs, such as "What if I am a bad parent?" or "What if the glass of wine that I had when I was pregnant caused all this?"

Still, I feel particularly sorry for regular educators who do not have any training regarding disabilities or behavioral modification strategies. According to several recent studies, the primary reason why regular education teachers leave the field early is because of the "problem" kids in their classes.

I believe it. I have given numerous workshops on how to teach students with ADHD. The regular educators who attend are almost always beaten down and emotionally drained. If raising five children was difficult for my mother, having five classes of twenty-five children is just as hard, especially when two of three of those children have ADHD, another two or three have learning disabilities, another two or three come from "troubled" homes, et cetera, et cetera, et cetera.

And then there are the siblings of children with ADHD. Many of them are just as stressed as the parents and teachers, if not more so. One little girl with whom I am working complains endlessly about her brother who has ADHD. Evidently, he constantly "bugs" her and never gives her "a moment alone." Moreover, he is frequently "in her things." For instance, she collects dolls, but he breaks them as quickly as she gets them. He will rip their heads off, cut their hair, and "feed" them to the dog. Plus, her parents "make" her play with him and then she gets blamed for whatever he does wrong.

It is hard enough being a kid today. It is even harder when you have to help raise a sibling who is out of control. I am sure that is how my brothers felt. Perhaps that is why they stayed away from me so much.

More needs to be done to help the people who are around children with ADHD. Regular educators need to be trained regarding disabling conditions and behavior modification strategies. Parents need to be given respite care and siblings need to be allowed to be children themselves.

Looking back, I can only guess how I affected my parents. At the very least, I tired them out and aged them beyond their years. At any rate, I know that they looked forward to spending time away from me. My mother, probably out of a need to have some quiet time, used to encourage me to go to bed as early as possible. She used to look at me, start to yawn, and say, "Wouldn't it feel good to be lying in your nice cool bed?" She would then yawn even more. That was all that it would take. For as much energy as I had, when it ran out, I would fall asleep right there on the spot. Unfortunately, as a result, I typically woke up before the crack of dawn. I still remember going down to the living room and watching the test patterns on the television. Since I was the only one awake, this was also when I did a lot of my worst damage.

Keep in mind that, as bad a kid as I was, I always wanted to be good. I always tried to do the right thing, but I usually did something to screw it up. Again, this is a common characteristic of kids with ADHD. Despite what the non-ADHD world thinks, people with ADHD don't usually do the things that we do on purpose. Actually, it is much more desirable to do what is expected and get along with everybody than it is to continually be an outcast and rejected. We want to be loved and accepted just like everybody else—but it just doesn't work out that way most of the time.

I remember that I used to stand over my parents as they slept. I didn't want to rouse them, so I would just stand over them waiting for them to wake up. Many times my mother was startled from a deep sleep only to find her youngest pride and joy breathing on her face.

After one such incident, I asked my mother if I could take apart a lamp. Being extremely tired and more than half asleep, she mumbled "all right" and rolled over. A couple hours later, she awoke and found me in the backyard with the lamp in several pieces on the picnic table. Needless to say, she wasn't happy. I would like to state for the record that I could have put the lamp back together again had I not chopped it up with a small hatchet.

As we discussed earlier, it wasn't just my parents who had to suffer. As with most siblings of children with ADHD, my brothers had their share of run-ins with me, especially the second-youngest and the middle child, Richard and John. Jim and Glenn are ten and eight years older than I am, so when I finally came along, they were doing their own things with their own friends. But Richard and John were only four and six years older than I, respectively. Plus, my mother used to make them play with me because nobody else would.

In retrospect, this was probably a bad idea. As much as I wanted to be with them, my brothers didn't want a thing to do with me. Any time that we were in close proximity for very long, some sort of altercation would ensue.

Richard and I, in particular, used to fight on a regular basis. They weren't really punching and kicking fights, although I did bite him in the back once. We were more like cats rolling around in the dirt. We would grab each other by the hair and tell each other "Let go!" To which the other would reply, "Not until you let go first!" And back and forth it would go as we pulled harder and harder.

I distinctly remember us grappling each other in the kitchen, yelling at the top of our lungs, "Let go! Let go! Let go!" I heard our father get up from his La-Z-Boy in the living room and start walking quickly toward us. The faster that he walked, the more trouble we were in. But we both refused to let go until the other did so first. Our father came into the room, grabbed us both by the hair or ear and dragged us upstairs to his bedroom where he had a tie rack full of belts. He then took one down and spanked us. Again, it was the 1970s; spanking was still all the rage.

Once, John, Richard, and I were lined up outside my father's bedroom door waiting for the leather to fall. If I recall correctly, we had either gotten into a fight or we couldn't stop giggling during dinner. Either way, we found ourselves standing in the hallway waiting for my father to select the proper belt, as we frequently did.

This particular time, Richard and John told me that I should put toilet paper down my pants so that the spanking wouldn't hurt so much. So, with my brothers smiling very broadly, I went into the bathroom and proceeded to unravel an entire roll and stuff the paper down the back of my pants. When it was my turn to "assume the position," my butt was three times its pre-spanked size. It looked like I had elephantiasis of the buttocks! I am not sure what upset my father more, the fact that I tried to pull one over on him or that I wasted an entire roll of toilet paper.

During another such lineup, my brothers convinced me that my father would only spank us until we cried. So I decided to start crying before he even selected the belt. I can still remember how red my father's face got. I can picture the frown that he had and how his eyes glared from behind his glasses. I remember him pulling me over his knees saying, "I'll give you something to cry about!"—which he did.

Another time, I was in the backyard playing with the hose. It was a hot summer day and I must have gotten some water on the roof of the garage because it was steaming. To me, it looked like smoke. So, without much difficulty, my brothers convinced me that I should try to put out the hidden fire while they went inside to call the fire department, which was only a block away.

About a half an hour passed. I was running around the garage, hosing it down so that the flames, which I couldn't see, didn't spread. Then my father pulled up. Seeing the now dripping garage and me with the hose, he stopped and shook his head. Suddenly it occurred to me that I probably was doing something wrong.

The moral of these stories is that I wasn't the brightest kid. Further, I routinely got in trouble, not because of anything I cooked up myself, but because I fell prey to other people's practical jokes. Of course, the fact that I rarely took the time to consider the consequences of my actions didn't help matters any.

This is another very common trait of people with ADHD. We tend to take things at face value—that is, when we pay attention to anything at all. I didn't question what my brothers told me basically because when I got something in my head, I did it. I couldn't stop myself. I was like a knee being tapped with a rubber hammer. My impulsivity baffled not only my family but myself as well.

My father grew tomatoes in the garden. He still does, actually. He has always been very proud of what he grows on his own. He would put his prizes on the windowsill in the kitchen until they ripened. He would then go around the neighborhood showing everybody how big and juicy the tomatoes were.

I remember walking by the kitchen table and seeing a knife. As the knife was flying from my hand, speeding toward the tomatoes, I thought to myself, "Now, that wasn't a very good idea"—which it wasn't. The knife would slam into the tomatoes sending a spray of tomato blood all over the windows. When he saw what I had done, my father would get furious!

What always stuns me is that this didn't just happen once or twice—it happened habitually. Many a piece of fruit died at the end of a thrown steak knife. Further, the words, "Now, that wasn't a very good idea" would echo in my head nearly as often as my mother saying "Jesus Christ, give me strength! You are such a rotten kid."

There are many more incidents involving my impulsivity. For instance, if I saw something that I wanted, I took it, sometimes without realizing it. Once I was in the grocery store with my mother. As I tried waiting patiently in line, I asked if I could have a candy bar. My mother said no, but somehow the candy bar ended up in my pocket anyway. I didn't consciously think about stealing it. I didn't plan on taking it. It just appeared in my pocket as if by magic! This happened more frequently than my parents realized.

Another time we were in the store and I begged my mother to buy some Jiffy Pop popcorn. I begged and begged and begged until she bought it just to shut me up. Back then, Jiffy Pop had this disposable pan with tinfoil over it. You were supposed to put the pan on the stove and the tinfoil would expand as the popcorn popped. I, however, couldn't wait. As soon as we got into the car, I ripped open the tinfoil looking for the popcorn, thus ruining it. I can still hear my mother sigh as she looked upward. All that aggravation and it got destroyed right away.

Of course, destruction was my middle name, although my brothers convinced me that it was really "Egghead." I remember sneaking downstairs one late Christmas Eve. My father was cursing as he tried to put

together some of my toys. I remember him saying, "I don't know why I
bother. He is just going to break them anyway." This was true. Toys
didn't last long with me. Christmas presents rarely lived long enough to
see the dawn of the New Year.

Once we went to Disneyland. I begged and begged and begged my
parents to let me get a hat that had the face of Donald Duck on it. When
you squeezed the bill of the cap, which was in the shape of a duck's bill,
it would quack. I broke the hat before we left the store. Of course, the
Disneyland trip was better known by Jergen historians for the dreaded
"Winnie the Pooh Incident."

As we walked around Disneyland, there were people dressed in cos-
tumes of various cartoon characters, such as Mickey Mouse and Goofy.
I saw some poor guy dressed as Winnie the Pooh and, for some reason,
I ran over to him as fast as I could go. Thinking that I was one of his
adoring fans, Winnie bent down to give me a hug. Much to his surprise,
I hauled off and hit him. It wasn't just one right hook to the face, but a
barrage of vicious blows to the prominent belly and several kicks to the
shin. To this day, I have a very vivid memory of a giant, golden-brown
bear trying to push me away with great fervor.

Of course, poor Santa Claus got his fair share too. I have several pictures of me as a child sitting on Santa's lap screaming. I am guessing that
this is probably a pretty typical reaction even from a normal kid. After
all, it is only natural for children to get a little freaked out when their
parents drop them on some stranger's lap, especially when the stranger
is covered with red fur and "ho, ho, ho-ing" like a lunatic. However,
while most kids might try to pull Santa's beard off, I went right for the
eyes. Again, I wasn't a pleasant child.

In addition to being dangerous to other people, my impulsive behavior was often potentially damaging to myself. Several times my lack of
impulse control put me in harm's way. Probably one of my most perilous
acts involved a can of Lysol and a book of matches.

I used to build models. Like playing with Legos or Lincoln Logs,
building models enabled me to have fun without the arduous task of
finding somebody who was willing to be around me. Once I built a
replica of the battleship USS *Missouri*. After the glue had dried, I filled
the bathtub with water and started floating my new toy.

Somehow, I got the idea that I could simulate a battle by flicking lit
matches at the ship. This seemed like a good idea at the time, so I sat

on the edge of the tub throwing flaming matches and watching the model burn. Then I heard somebody come into the house. Realizing that my parents probably would not like what I was doing, I submerged the smoldering boat and sprayed Lysol all over the bathroom. I nearly empted the entire can in an effort to cover up the stench from the burning plastic.

As soon as I heard the person leave, I put the boat back in the tub and, without thinking, flicked another match. Suddenly, for a sliver of a second, I was engulfed in flames. Ribbons of fire appeared wherever I had sprayed the Lysol. Flames raced up the walls and licked the ceiling. They danced on the water in the tub. I must have gotten some Lysol on me because my hands and arms blazed brightly. Then everything was fine. The Lysol had burned away and the flames disappeared.

Very calmly, I took the model to my bedroom, sat on the bed, and started shaking. Fortunately, I wasn't hurt and nothing was damaged. But my poor judgment could have burnt the house down with me along with it.

The weeks leading up to the Fourth of July were particularly precarious. My brothers and the neighborhood children loved fireworks. We all did. Back then it was very easy to get firecrackers with remarkable power. There were M-80s and similar explosives that could blow huge holes in ground, as well as fingers from hands.

Once I was playing with some older kids who lived up the street. They had a bag full of pyrotechnics of almost every design. They gave me an M-80 to throw off their back porch. But just as they lit it, I got distracted. Somebody was doing something interesting that caught my eye. The kid who lit the explosive was yelling at me to "Throw it! Throw it!" but I wasn't paying attention. I was just standing there with a small piece of dynamite in my hand. The kid knocked the M-80 from my grasp and threw me to the ground. It exploded a few feet away leaving a high-pitched ringing in my ears that I thought would never go away.

Another time we were shooting off bottle rockets and again my impulsivity got the best of me. Trying to be funny, I grabbed a bottle rocket, lit it, and pointed at the back of somebody's head. Just as it shot out of my hand, the boy turned around and saw what I was doing. He tried to dive out of the way but there was no time. The bottle rocket grazed his left temple and exploded a fraction of a second later. Had it exploded on impact, he probably would have lost an eye.

Because of incidents like these, I developed at a pretty young age a kind of inner voice. Actually, as we will discuss later, I had several inner voices all talking to me at the same time. It was, and is, maddening at times.

One voice in particular would ask me "What are you doing wrong?" This voice would become especially loud whenever I heard my father's car pull into the driveway. As soon as my father or mother would come home, I would stop whatever I was doing and think to myself, "What am I doing wrong?" Usually, I would be doing something bad, like jumping on the bed, or I had forgotten to do something that I was supposed to do.

Something that I frequently forgot to do was take the trash out. This was my family chore to perform. I think trash days were on Wednesdays. So on Tuesday nights, I was supposed to take the two metal trashcans from the back of the house and place them by the curb. Then, when I got home from school the next day, I was supposed to take the empty cans back behind the house.

No matter how hard I tried, I simply could not remember to do these two simple tasks. It was almost as if my mind could not retain the fact that I was expected to do something important Tuesday nights and Wednesday afternoons. Nearly every week, my father was beside himself with anger.

Once I was lying on the floor of the living room, watching television. My father walked in and told me to put the garbage out. I remember getting up to one knee, determined to do as my father asked before he got any angrier. But something on the television caught my eye and I laid back down on the floor.

It seemed like only seconds passed. To me, my father had just walked in and told me to get the trashcans to the curb and I was about to do it. Then I felt the familiar sting of my father's hand whacking me on the back of my head. "What did I tell you? Get the goddamned garage cans out front," he yelled. I remember how shocked I was to see that it was already dark outside. He had told me to get the trashcans out several hours before but, to me, it seemed like just a few minutes, if not seconds, had passed.

Another time I was in the kitchen eating after getting home from school. My father came in from work and asked me if I had brought the trashcans back from the curb. Without thinking about it, I must have said that I had, kind of like an unconscious, spur-of-the-moment response that was so typical of me. My father grabbed me by the ear, pulled me to the curb, put his glasses on my face, and then shoved my head into the trashcans that were waiting to be taken back behind the house.

This is how things went for me. For the most part, I really tried to be a good kid. I really did. Honest! I know it sounds like I was just being obnoxious on purpose, but I really wasn't trying to be. I wanted nothing more than to be loved and accepted. I wanted to be as smart, athletic, liked, and funny as my brothers. I really tried to be a good person. I tried to do what I was told and to behave myself. It was just that, the harder I tried, the worst things got and the angrier people became.

Moreover, my behavior was frequently beyond my control. I did things that I didn't even realize I had done. It was like I would black out and then wake up standing in the ruins caused by my impulses, or that I was Dr. Jekyll and I was getting blamed for everything that Mr. Hyde was doing.

For instance, I went through a period of sighing melodramatically. I think I got that from my father. Whenever I did something wrong, he would take off his glasses, shake his head, look at me, and let loose this heavy sigh that dripped with disgust.

For a while, I adopted the same sigh. I remember that I was sitting on the sofa reading. My father told me to do something, probably for the third or fourth time. I sighed deeply. My father pointed his finger at me and said, "You sigh like that again and I will smack you across your mouth." Well, I must have sighed again because, true to his word, my father turned around and backhanded me across the cheek. I remember sitting there frozen, wondering what I did to deserve being slapped. Then I realized that I had just sighed again.

So that was my life growing up. I was constantly causing a nuisance. If I didn't do something wrong, I would forget to do what I was told or I would say something that would get me smacked. Soon, I began to live in constant fear that I would do or say something that would get me in trouble. As you will see, I am plagued by the same feelings to this very day.

3

SEND IN THE TEACHERS

The beginning of my formal education was not easy for me. This is pretty predictable for people with ADHD. Prior to entering school, children are not forced to remain seated for long periods of time. They can run and jump around outside, expelling all of their pent-up energy. They also don't have to complete academic tasks by a certain deadline or concentrate on minute details.

After entering school, on the other hand, children suddenly have to sit down and follow numerous, often arbitrary, rules—such as raising your hand before speaking and staying in your seat. They also have to share the attention of the adult with twenty other children. Consequently, going to school often extenuates the problems that children with ADHD have regarding their hyperactivity, impulsivity, and inattention. In fact, in many cases, it isn't until school starts that symptoms of ADHD become readily apparent or severe enough to draw concern.

It should be noted that if a child goes to school, is fine, and then starts exhibiting symptoms later on in life, she or he probably doesn't actually have ADHD. As we discussed in the introduction, people do not "develop" or "get" ADHD. Their symptoms might worsen or lessen depending upon their environment, but they don't just suddenly become hyperactive, inattentive, or impulsive overnight. If they do, they have some other condition, such as seizures or drug problems.

At any rate, the first few years of formal education tend to be crucial when identifying kids with ADHD. This is not to say that people, such as myself, can't be diagnosed later on. They can. I was in my twenties when I was diagnosed. Still, according to the accepted definition of ADHD, some symptoms have to be evident by age seven. This means that teachers, especially those at the early levels, hold particular insight as to whether a child might or might not have ADHD. After all, they have a great deal of experience and a diverse comparison group.

Unlike any of my brothers, I went to preschool. I think that the main purpose of preschool was to give my mother a break from my challeng-ing behavior. At that time, my mother was a stay-at-home mom. Being stuck in the same house with me all alone all day must have been very grueling for her. At least when my older brothers were around, I had somebody else to pester and watch me. Now that they were in school, the sensible thing for my mother to do was to palm me off on some other poor, unsuspecting adult.

Initially, the preschool was a positive experience. After one of the first days, I came home all excited and announced that I was the "smartest boy in the class!" Not surprisingly, things quickly went downhill from there. Day after day, my enthusiasm for school declined, a trend that would continue for the next eighteen years.

I constantly got into trouble, although I didn't mean to. I simply could not follow the rules no matter how hard I tried. For instance, off to the side of the preschool room were cubbies where we were to put our coats and other belongings. For whatever reason, I either frequently forgot or refused to put my stuff away. In fact, I can still vaguely picture a woman standing over me and shaking her finger in disapproval of my "poor attitude."

Also in the room was a story rug. Here we sat every day at a prede-termined time and listened to one of the teachers read us a story. I used to sit on the far edge of the story rug, but I would have great difficulty keeping still. I would fidget, look around, get up, and eventually wander off to other parts of the room.

At first, the teachers continued their scoldings, but that didn't work. I was moved to the front of the rug where they could quickly redirect my attention, but I kept getting distracted by the kids who were sitting behind me. They then made me sit by my cubby; however, just as I was not able to remain seated on the story rug, I wasn't able to sit still by my cubby either. Finally the teachers had had enough.

To this day, my mother finds great pleasure in telling the story about how the nice old ladies from the preschool called her one morning. They apparently were beside themselves and informed my mother that I wasn't cooperating. They then asked for her permission to spank me. As I mentioned earlier, my mother is a Norwegian-Swedish American. She didn't believe in spanking, but she was quite familiar with how taxing I was and how hard it was to control me. So, reluctantly, she gave her consent.

When I came home that day, my mother looked down at me and asked, "Are you going to start cooperating?" The way my mother tells it, I looked back up at her and said in a very sad, four-year-old voice, "I cooperate." Those teachers might have warmed my butt, but they didn't break my spirit! I had more in store for them!

The preschool was at the back of a church. I don't know if the preschool was actually church-affiliated or whether the school was merely renting space. In any case, the teachers certainly were not nuns or else they might have lost their faith in God after working with me.

Shortly after the spanking incident, I made a break for it. When nobody was looking, I ran from the preschool and into the church part of the building. I can still recall hiding under a pew as teachers walked from room to room calling my name and promising me a piece of candy if I would come back.

The funny thing is that I returned on my own pretty quickly. Not because I wanted any candy. I wasn't that easy. I basically got bored crouching under the pew. I probably thought the whole affair was funny for three or four seconds and then had to find something else that would hold my attention.

The same thing happened when I ran away from home. Well, I really didn't run far. I crawled underneath the porch. After a minute or two had passed, and nobody made an effort to locate me, I left my hiding place and resumed my terrorizing. The little monster would not be ignored—nor was he very patient.

My attention span severely limited my chances at becoming a professional hide-and-go-seek player. I would find really good spots in which to hide, but I didn't have the patience to remain there for very long. Further, I slowly started wondering if my brothers were actually trying to find me. Once, I hid in the basement and got bored. When I went back upstairs, I found that the door was barricaded shut by several kitchen chairs.

Kindergarten wasn't much better than preschool. In my mind's eye, my teacher, Mrs. Roush, was ancient. She had most, if not all, of my brothers in her classes at one time or another. I recall her being very nice and kind. In fact, she was one of the few educators who didn't express a great deal of distress about my behavior. In a note to my mother she only said, "Robbie certainly has more energy than did his brothers."

The academic portion of kindergarten, such as it was, didn't bother me. From the paperwork that I still have, Mrs. Roush found me to be very bright, but I was, as she said, "socially behind." I also had difficulty playing well with others. Specifically, I got easily frustrated when things didn't go my way and would start crying at the drop of a hat. Further, I didn't pick up my toys or put my things away and I had to be constantly prompted to follow the rules. Still, I was recommended to continue on to first grade.

Even more so than kindergarten, elementary school was exasperating for me. Again, it wasn't the academics. Although I didn't get stellar grades, this was mainly due to uncompleted work and careless mistakes, not because I didn't understand the material. My most pressing problem involved my social skills, or lack of them.

Growing up in Beach Grove, I lived on Lane Place. You couldn't have asked for a better street on which to grow up. Lane Place was a block long and the only people who would drive down it were either residents or the occasional driver who somehow got turned around and lost. Traffic, therefore, was minimal.

Further, Lane Place was centrally located. Only a couple blocks away was downtown Beach Grove where there were many shops, including a movie theater, pet store, an old fashioned mom-and-pop candy shop, and a bowling alley with the latest in video games, such as Space Invaders and Asteroids. Lane Place was also close to a forest preserve where I used to ride my bike.

The best thing about Lane Place was that there were tons of kids around. Even twenty-five years later, I can name a couple dozen of my classmates who lived within a block of us. During the summer nights, the street was usually full of children playing whiffle ball, tag, Mr. Wolf what time is it, and a variety of other games.

Despite the overwhelming number of potential playmates and the size of my family, I was extremely lonely as a child. I remember looking down on the street from my bedroom window, watching the hordes of children running here and there. Laughing. Playing. Have a good time. I, on the other hand, felt very dark and empty and angry.

Even at such a young age, I was getting incredibly frustrated. I wanted to be social and play with the other kids, but I couldn't. I couldn't tolerate following their stupid rules, and waiting for them to take their turn was excruciatingly painful for me. The other kids didn't move fast enough and whenever I tried to speed things up, they got upset. It made me want to scream.

That was another problem that I had. The other kids didn't understand me and I didn't understand them. I would say whatever popped into my head and they would get upset. Or I would bounce from one topic to another and they couldn't figure out what I was talking about. So they just assumed that I was an idiot and treated me as such. After even brief interactions, I usually went home either angry or crying.

Another reason why I didn't play much with the other children was because I had asthma. For a few years, it was pretty bad. I had to go to the hospital more than once. As soon as I started wheezing, my mother would make me come in and sit in my air-conditioned bedroom. There, I sat by the window and watched the fun from a distance.

It is interesting to note that my pediatrician used to think that my hyperactivity and inattentiveness was caused by my asthma medicine. As a matter of fact, the medicine was later taken off the market. Evidently it caused some sort of heath problems in kids.

Whether it was because of my asthma, poor attention span, impulsive behavior, or general lack of athletic ability, I just was not very good at most games. My brother Richard and I used to play whiffle ball, but I never won and I got very upset when he did his "victory lap" around the house. Moreover, except for our next-door neighbors, Chrissy and Nancy, nobody seemed terribly interested in being with me. Why be with me when they could be with Richard or John, both of whom were very fun and had better social skills than I had?

Because of my social isolation, I tended to play by myself. I played with Legos, Lincoln Logs, and erector sets—anything that allowed me to use my hands. I also used to write a lot. I had notebooks full of stupid stories with recurring characters, such as "Buck Jergen," a take-off of Buck Rogers, and "James Rich," a private investigator who solved all kinds of mysterious crimes.

I spent most of my time with the various animals in my life. There was our dog Whiskers, our neighbors' dogs Buffy and Fluffy, and a herd of gerbils that my mother let me buy. I also spent a lot of time alone in the nearby forest preserve watching the birds, squirrels, and the occasional deer. The nice thing about animals is that they don't make fun of the idiotic things that you do. They don't judge or call you stupid. They just sit and listen to all of your problems as if they were their own.

As I was growing up, animals played a huge part of my life. I told them everything. They listened and didn't tease me. They didn't say, "Jesus Christ, give me strength! You are such a rotten kid!" They didn't shake their head and sigh when they looked at me. They didn't lock me in closets or the basement. They didn't spank me because I couldn't sit still. They accepted me for who I was.

Just as I didn't play very much with the kids around Lane Place, I didn't play much with my peers at Hillside Elementary School. It wasn't that I was unpopular or that I was hated. Actually, kids with ADHD tend to be the center of attention. We are a good source of entertainment for everybody—that is, for everybody except the teachers.

I remember many times when other children would encourage me to do things that would get me in trouble. For example, when Becky Webster was about to sit down, Forrest Wager told me to pull her chair out from underneath her. I did and Becky fell sprawling on the floor.

This was a pretty age-appropriate prank. The problem was that I didn't know when to stop. I would keep pulling the same stunt well after it stopped being funny. I must have pulled Becky's chair out from underneath her a dozen times. The last time, she cracked her head on a table and had to go to the nurse's office. To this day, I still feel bad about that.

While I was well known because of my antics and last name, not many people wanted me around when the serious playing had to be done. I was rarely picked to be on the kickball teams during recess. Instead, I always had to keep score or be an umpire, if I was allowed to be involved at all.

More often than not, I would wander around the playground, walking from group to group, hoping that somebody would talk to or play with me. It wasn't that I didn't want to play with the other kids. I did—desperately. But I didn't know how to interact or initiate conversations. I never knew what to say or when to say it. For me, joining a group of kids was much like a blind person trying to skip rope. I never knew when to jump in. Sometimes there would be a lull in the conversation and I would bring up something new, such as the fact that I had just seen a good movie or something. The other kids would look rather annoyed and go back to whatever they were talking about. Eventually, I would wander away.

Looking back, I can see the first seed of depression growing. However, I wasn't completely sullen. I was still able to crack jokes and be funny—usually at the most inappropriate times.

Rather than look like the odd man out during recess, I started hiding in the bathroom. I would bring a comic book into the stall, lock the door, and read until I heard the bell ring and the cheerful voices of my classmates come back into the building. A very grim darkness was falling on me, but the worst was yet to come.

I don't remember much from elementary school, but I do recall one incident very clearly. I was standing at the front of the classroom, staring blankly at the fish tank, when Barbara Bannow walked up to me, made a snide comment, and then ran away. She literally ran out of the room and down the hallway, leaving me standing there rather hurt and perplexed.

I ran into Barb when we were in our twenties. We were chatting about the "old times" when she brought up that event. "Do you remember the time by the fish tank and I ran away?" she asked. Of course I did, it was one of those things that always puzzled me. "Well," she said, "some of the other kids bet me that I couldn't get the last word with you. So I decided to say something and then run."

That conversation, as we sat in a park nearly twenty years after the fact, was extremely enlightening for me. You see, at the time I always felt that I was invisible, that nobody knew that I existed, except when I was being yelled at. But Barb gave me her perspective and the perspective of the other kids in our class.

"You were always strange," she told me. "Not in a bad way," she added reassuringly. "Just different. You would always have something odd to say, something completely out of the blue that would leave us scratching our heads. We never knew what you were talking about or whether your comments were meant as put-downs or if you were just being silly. A lot of us just didn't know how to take you."

To this day, Barb's insights epitomized my relationship with other people. As you will soon see, my entire life has been one social faux pas after another. Even now, I am not very good with people and frequently find myself apologizing for what I say and do.

At the time, my elementary school teachers didn't seem to notice my isolation. Perhaps they were more concerned about my in-class behavior, which was steadily getting more and more disruptive. Almost on a weekly basis, I was asked to sit in the hallway. Sometimes when I got off the bus in the morning, my desk and chair would already be waiting for me by the lockers.

Once my sixth-grade teacher, Ms. Jackson, called me over to her desk before class started and handed me a yardstick. She asked me to go measure around the school and then come back to report my findings. She didn't mean just around the school building, but the entire school grounds. Around the playground, the loading dock, the front lawn, the ball diamonds—all around the *entire* school.

I was more than happy to do so. I hated being in class. So, I took the yardstick and measured. It took me a couple hours, but I was able to get a rough estimate of how many yards it was around the school.

When I came back, I told her my results. Ms. Jackson smiled and handed me another stick. She then instructed me to go back outside and do the same thing, but this time using a meter.

Again, I was very happy to "cooperate." I liked being outside by myself, crawling around the edge of the school. By the end of the day, I came back into class and reported my second findings. Not only did this activity get me out of class but it was also very educational. I now know that a meter is either bigger or smaller than a yard!

Over the years, my mother has kept all of her notes from various parent-teacher meetings. She also kept my report cards, which have comments from teachers written on the back. Reading them now reveals some very interesting information. They also make me feel a bit sad. Here is what they had to say.

Kindergarten, Mrs. Roush:

A note to my mother indicates that I was able to "listen with a purpose" but it "depends upon who is near him." Apparently, I was very distractible. Mrs. Roush also stated that I "could improve putting materials away" and that I didn't "use work-play time constructively." An interesting comment scribbled on the bottom of a report says that I "tolerated" others. Not that I "got along" with others. Not that I "played well" with others, but that I "tolerated" others. Further, she said that I had a "good disposition."

First Grade, Miss Dill:

On my first report card, the "needs improvement" box was checked for "Is orderly and neat," "Speaks clearly," "Writes legibly," "Forms letters correctly," and "Uses neatness in writing." Miss Dill also wrote, "Robby needs to concentrate more on the work at hand. He is in too big of a hurry, which leads to unnecessary mistakes and messiness. With a little effort and maturation on his part, I am sure he will have greater success during the last half of the year."

At the end of the year, Ms. Dill wrote, "Robby is improving but still needs work in reading and math. With effort on his part, I am sure he can meet his academic needs." In the materials that my mother saved, there is a very thoughtful note from Ms. Dill to me saying, "I will always remember you, Robert, as someone who tires very hard."

Yes, I tried hard, particularly when I was young. But it seems clear from her notes that my effort wasn't paying off. Later teachers would make the same observations.

Second Grade, Ms. Sweeney:

At the end of the first semester of second grade, Ms. Sweeney wrote, "Rob is having difficulties with phonics—particularly vowels. He tries to read too quickly and tends to make word substitutions. He has been working very hard to improve his handwriting. He is having some problems with fractions but his other math skills are good. I am pleased with Rob's attitudes towards his work."

Note that yet another teacher indicated that I tried and that I had a good attitude. I wasn't just goofing off or overtly trying to upset my teachers. I was trying to be a good kid. I was doing my work too fast, but at least I was trying to do it. I apparently made careless mistakes, which is typical of kids with ADHD. Also note the problems with phonics. This will be explained later in my life.

On my end-of-the-year report card, Ms. Sweeney just indicated that, "He is having some difficulty with irregular vowel spellings." There is also a note from a parent-teacher meeting that says, "Rob does not put forth good effort or makes wise use of his time."

By the second part of second grade, things appear to have started to change. I was still making careless mistakes and having problems with sounds, but I apparently was starting to give up. This trend continued for many years to come.

Third Grade, Ms. Miller:

On my report card, Ms. Miller indicated that I needed improvement "using correct spelling in written work" and "showing accuracy in computations." At the end of the first term, she wrote, "Robert has been trying very hard. His reading is improving though he ignores contractions and doesn't know some of them. He tends to substitute small words or say just any word that comes to his mind that begins with the same sound. Perhaps this is a bit of carelessness. He is not always accurate in his math papers though he seems to understand the basic concept. This again is probably carelessness. He seems slightly immature and this can produce carelessness."

Here I at least started to try again. However, I made the same mistakes as I did the previous two grades. Accuracy was an ongoing problem, and will be for many years to come. It wasn't that I didn't understand what to do, I just was very careless and rushed through my work, as several teachers had already stated.

At the end of my third grade, Ms. Miller wrote, "Rob has improving a bit in reading. He seems more interested in it. He needs to learn his 8's and 9's in multiplication. His cursive is more legible but he needs to remember to cross t's and dot i's. Also, he needs to remember punctuating rules when writing. It is a pleasure to have Rob in class."

A note to my mother says, "Robert is very active and is eager to get his work done. He sometimes does not hear sounds too well and I think it hinders his sounding out words both in reading and spelling. He reads aloud rather 'choppily' and seems insecure."

By the end of third grade, I was still having problems with details. Ms. Miller's comment that I was "very active" is probably teacher-parent code for "Your kid drives me crazy!" It is interesting to see how my hyperactivity not only affected my in-class behavior but also my academics—especially my math and reading.

Fourth Grade, Ms. Fiene:

We started getting letter grades in fourth grade. For the first semester, I got a C− in reading, C in language arts, B in mathematics, C in social studies, and B in science. Ms. Fiene wrote that, "Robert can do better in school. He is having some difficulty because he has been sick." She also indicated that I was not neat and that my desk was "in disarray."

For the second semester, I got a B− in reading, C in language arts, B in mathematics, C in social studies, and a C in science. Ms. Fiene wrote, "Robert seems to be enjoying school more. He needs to put forth more effort." A note to my mother indicated that my penmanship was sloppy and that "Robert tries hard but is having some difficulties with his work. He appears to be trying."

Whether I was really trying or not is unclear. I remember fourth grade and I don't think that I tried very hard. In fact, I was starting to give up again, as my frequent absences illustrate.

Fifth Grade, Ms. Kierznowski:

In fifth grade, I got all B−'s with the exception of a C in reading. My teacher wrote, "In math some of my concern is careless errors. He seems to understand the concepts but makes mistakes in the computations."

Yet another teacher, the fifth in five years, indicated that I have a problem with being careless. Reading continued to be a problem for me.

Sixth Grade, Ms. Jackson:

In sixth grade, I got mostly Cs. Ms. Jackson wrote that I needed improvement in "Shows self-confidence," "Is orderly and neat," and "Uses time wisely." She also sent a note home saying that "More participation in class discussions would not only help Rob develop concepts but would benefit his classmates." There are also notes on several homework assignments complaining about my spelling and penmanship.

Ms. Jackson is the teacher who had me measure around the school. She also had me go read underneath a big tree on the playground while everybody else sat inside. More than any other teacher, she seemed to realize that I had a problem, but she dealt with it by removing me from the class.

This data illustrates a pattern of behavior that was well documented before I even completed first grade. I clearly had problems paying attention. Numerous teachers indicated that I rushed through work, missed details, made careless mistakes, especially in math and reading, and that I was messy. Several teachers also said that I was socially immature.

Also notice the progression of the grades from mainly Bs to mostly Cs. This will be the beginning of a downward trend that will continue throughout junior high and high school. Further, as Ms. Fiene stated, I was missing more and more school as I got older. She said that I was "sick." In reality, I was faking it most of the time. By third grade, I hated going to school and frequently told my mother that I was too ill to go. Moreover, when I did show up, I would often go to the nurse's office and pretend to have a headache. She would let me lie down for a half hour or so and then make me go back to class. Still, I was more than happy to get out of class for even part of the day.

Perhaps most important is the comment that Ms. Fiene wrote after the second semester of fourth grade. She noted that I appeared to be "enjoying school more," implying that I was noticeably depressed during the first semester. Ms. Jackson in sixth grade also was concerned about my participation, suggesting that I was more withdrawn than she liked.

Ms. Fiene's and Ms. Jackson's comments are significant because they indicate a change in my behavior and outlook. Earlier teachers, such as Mrs. Roush, Miller, and Dill, found that I was social and personable. They actually wrote very positive comments, such as that it was a pleasure to have me in class and that I was a "joy." These might have been just stock phases made to make parents feel good; however, the change in me seems to be very noticeable. By the time sixth grade ended, my grades were down, I was not participating in class, and I no longer described as a happy child. The worst was just around the corner.

4

JUNIOR HIGH: HEROES AND HOPE GONE

Around fifth grade, I had a small handful of friends. There was Mike Stone, Steve Pollock, and Mark Chester. Mark was the cute one, Steve was the quiet one, Mike was the cuddly one, and I was the dark, gloomy, emotional one. Together, we referred to ourselves as "The Beatles"; Mark was Paul McCartney, Mike was Ringo Starr, Steve was George Harrison, and I was John Lennon.

I was exposed to the Beatles by my brothers, especially Richard and John. They had all of their records and played them regularly. Part of me was into the Beatles because I wanted to be like my brothers, but there was something else attracting me to them.

There was something about John Lennon that really appealed to me. It still does; I remain a big fan. To me, Lennon seemed so brooding and deep, yet intelligent and witty. In him I saw a little of myself as well as a lot of who I wanted to be.

I entered O'Neill Junior High School in August 1980. On December 7 of that year, John Lennon was murdered outside his home in New York. His death devastated me. I remember coming out of my bedroom to get ready to go to school and seeing my mother in the hallway. She told me that Lennon had been killed the night before. I didn't react right away. I stepped back into my bedroom, closed my door, and sat down on my bed. After a couple of minutes staring at the wall, I started bawling my eyes out. I still get upset thinking about it. Junior high started out very difficult and it was about to get worse.

While Mike, Mark, Steve, and I hung out periodically during fifth grade, by the end of sixth grade, we rarely saw each other. When I went into junior high, I had no friends, at least nobody that I went out with or spoke to on a regular basis. Whereas recess in elementary school was uncomfortable for me, lunch and passing periods during junior high were absolutely horrid.

During passing periods, kids stood around and talked. They would gather at the stairwells and swap stories. They would pass notes, talk about the people they had crushes on, and make fun of anybody who was different.

I was different. My days of feeling invisible were gone. I now felt like I had a big spotlight on me, an X on my forehead, or maybe a bull's-eye on my back. As I approached the stairwells, my heart would pound. My mouth would go dry. My armpits would rain with sweat. I was afraid that people would say something or make fun of me. Sometimes they did. Sometimes they didn't.

It wasn't cool to get to class early, but I had no place else to go. I tried hiding in the bathrooms, but that was where the "bad kids" were, the smokers or druggies. I wasn't welcome in their world. Once I went in to use the bathroom and they pushed me out the door. I had no safe place to be. In the end, I would just sit in class by myself while all the other kids laughed and joked in the hallways.

Lunch was even worse. Whereas passing periods only lasted ten or fifteen minutes, lunch dragged on for nearly an hour. It was forty-five minutes of anxiety-ridden hell.

Usually, I sat by myself in the corner. Sometimes I sat with a kid nicknamed "Froggie" who had Down syndrome and was in special education. People noticed and made fun of me, but I didn't have much of a choice. I had to eat and the teachers wouldn't let kids out of the lunchroom until the period had ended. For me, it never ended fast enough.

Weekends were also really tough for me. By the early 1980s, my oldest brothers, Jim and Glenn, were in college and pretty much out of the picture. Richard and John were in high school. Further, they were all dating and had their own lives, so we didn't interact much anymore.

Each weekend, Rich and John had friends come over or they would go out with some attractive girl. My parents played bridge at the neighbor's house. And I sat all alone at home watching television. I watched *The Love Boat*, *Fantasy Island*, and *Saturday Night Live*. After *Saturday Night Live*, I cried myself to sleep.

During junior high, a new beast reared its terrifying head—a monster that frightens me to this very day. I was starting to be attracted to girls. Unfortunately, being the youngest of five boys, I had no experience with females. What was even worse, I had no social skills and was seen as immature by everybody around me. While being a Jergen gave me a certain degree of popularity, I was skinny and very gawky. I was so skinny that I used to wear sweatpants underneath my jeans so that it would look like I had a butt.

My problems with women are legendary. I didn't have my first date until I was a sophomore in high school and then not again until I was a senior and then not again until my sophomore year in college. As we will discuss later in great detail, I have been hung up on by more women than a telemarketer.

During seventh and eighth grades, however, girls had yet to do their damage. I was interested, but too shy to approach anybody for a date. And nobody was interested in me. Meanwhile, my academic difficulties that began in elementary school continued to spiral out of control.

In seventh grade, I got all Cs, with the exception of a B in physical education and a B in mathematics. The comments made by my teachers mirror what was said throughout the six previous years. Mr. Gorski, my reading teacher, wrote, "I am a little disappointed. Rob, with more effort, could easily have done much better." Mrs. Wilson, my science teacher wrote, "Rob is slow about making up late work." Finally, Mrs. Dymond, my English teacher, said that I needed to study more and "turn in daily assignments."

Of my six academic teachers that I had that year, four indicated that I didn't turn in my homework on time, three said that I didn't use class time well, and two said that I didn't perform well on tests. Further, I was absent from school eighteen times during the school year. I wonder how many of these I actually was sick.

If my parents and Mr. Gorski were disappointed in my grades in seventh grade, they would be shocked at my performance the following year.

I got Bs in English and physical education and Cs in reading and mathematics. Unfortunately, I got Ds in science and social studies. As far as I know, these were the first Ds that any of the Jergen boys had ever gotten. Comments from my teachers highlight some of my difficulties.

My home economics teacher said that I was "<u>usually</u> cooperative" but that I talked too much and said inappropriate things (note that "usually" was underlined twice). My mathematics teacher said that I had earned a low C and that "daily work still needs improvement. Too many assignments are missing." My reading teacher wrote, "C minus. Rob's many absences have caused him to fall behind in his daily work. Rob could have gotten a B with a little more effort." My social studies teacher wrote, "Rob was doing well the first half of the trimester, he was earning a B. The second half he did not apply himself. He was negligent in completing several assignments and failed the last test." Finally, my English teacher wrote, "Rob would have made a B if he had made up all the work that he missed." Moreover, nearly all of my teachers checked the boxes indicating that I didn't perform to my ability, make a consistent effort, follow directions, make up missed assignments, or use class time effectively.

On the back of my report card for physical education, there are two important handwritten entries. The first is mine. It is barely legible and nearly every third word is misspelled. I wrote, "My ability in most of the sports was fair. Basketball was the worst. My behavior was good at all times. I really don't know why I got a B. My behavior was good. I helped out a lot. I guess I didn't get an A because I didn't always bring my gym suit." This was true. I frequently forgot my gym suit at home.

The second note is from my mother. It simply says, "All I ask is that you participate." I can still hear her disappointment. I can also sense her frustration. Looking back, I know that everybody was worried about me, although I didn't realize it at the time.

My grades were getting worse and worse and my personality was changing. The latter was more than just typical adolescence, although that was probably causing part of my extreme moodiness. The depression that started around fifth grade was now weighing heavier upon me and becoming more pronounced.

I often found myself wandering around alone. Almost in a trance, I walked to my old elementary school a couple miles away and the church where I went to preschool. It is very hard to explain, but it felt like I was looking for something. I would sit on the playground equipment and try to see things that weren't there anymore. I went through a period of uncontrollable crying. I would burst into tears for no reason. Then I started to feel nothing. Nothing at all. I was numb.

As far back as I can remember, I always had a certain view of my future. It was very much like a premonition or, perhaps, foreshadowing. I pictured myself in a white padded room with bright white lights. I would be wearing a straitjacket and sitting in the corner. At first, my family would come see me every day. Then, my parents would come on the weekends. Then only on holidays. Eventually, they would stop coming altogether.

Oddly, the certainty that I was eventually going to go insane didn't provoke any bad feelings. Quite the contrary—it made me feel better, much better actually. The idea of going crazy was like slipping on a warm and familiar sweatshirt or lying in a hot bathtub on a cold day. I was actually looking forward to it. Being put into a psychiatric ward would mean that I would no longer have to struggle with my day-to-day existence. I would no longer have to watch what I said. I would no longer have to strain to pay attention. I would no longer have to force myself to sit still or not to act on my many bizarre impulses, such as my strong desires to pull fire alarms, pat girls on the butt, or poke people in the nose with my finger.

As I wandered aimlessly around, I began thinking about killing myself. To tell you the truth, since elementary school, the thought of death regularly popped into my thoughts. I think to some people I was, and still am, a little morbid. During a Thanksgiving dinner, I blurted out, "I want to be cremated after I die." My family just glanced at me and kept eating.

Throughout junior high, my depression got more acute. I had very few friends, and nobody with whom I could talk openly. My grades were plummeting. I kept doing things that made me an outcast. I felt awkward, stupid, and very much alone. Perhaps the hardest thing involved church.

My family was Lutheran. They were, but I wasn't. I hated going to church and I hated going to Sunday school and confirmation class even more. It wasn't that I didn't believe in all of these wonderful ideas that they were trying to teach us. Actually, finding a higher purpose, or a God who loved me for who I was, was exactly what I needed. But the other kids made fun of me. They were cruel and mean. They would make fun of what I wore or my big teeth or the fact that I didn't know what we were doing in class. I sat in the last row of tables, in the corner. A good day was when nobody spoke to me.

Of course there were reasons why the kids made fun of me. I would blurt out things and ask questions that they felt were stupid. I also had huge problems paying attention. I couldn't follow along when they were reading from the Bible and I never knew what was happening. There were times when I couldn't read when called on. My mind was in utter chaos and my behavior seemed to be as well. I felt so badly that I started hiding in the bathroom, much as I did during recess in elementary school. I brought a comic book and hid. Then I would stand in front of the church and wait for my parents to pick me up. I would tell them that class ended early and that everybody else had gone home already.

Sometimes, I would try missing church by taking an extra-long shower. My father would pound on the bathroom door and I would pretend not to hear him. He wasn't happy, but it was a lot better than going to church. I wasn't treated well by the pastors or my peers. Plus, I soon stopped believing in God. I simply couldn't believe that such a cruel being could exist.

Finally, I decided to take a stand. I told my parents that I wasn't going to church anymore. If they were not happy before, they were now absolutely fuming. They yelled at me. They threatened me. They scorned me. They did everything they could to make me go, but I refused. Eventually, they agreed to let me drop out if I went to talk to the pastor.

I remember that day very well. My father brought me to speak with the pastor who tried convincing me that I was making a horrible mistake. But I held firm and told him that I didn't believe in God. After a much one-sided discussion, he told me to wait in the next room.

While in the next room, I listened up against the door. The pastor was now talking to my father. I remember my father saying, "We just don't know what to do with him." He repeated that twice. I felt like crying, but I had run out of tears.

On the way home from my meeting with the pastor, my father said in a very quiet voice, "You are making your mother very upset." He didn't speak to me again for four days. Even now, my brothers bring up the fact that I am going to hell and that I am a "heathen."

The growing isolation from my family caused by refusal to go to church, as well as my social and academic ineptness, took its toll. I kept waiting for the day that I would be put in the white padded room. I kept waiting, but it wasn't coming quickly enough. Finally, I made a decision.

The Scholzes moved to Lane Place when their youngest daughter, Nancy, was an infant. Nancy and I grew up together. For many years, when we were younger, we were inseparable. We did everything together. She was, and is, the closest thing that I had to a sister. She and her family are still very much a part of my life. I love them as if they were biological relatives. By the time we were in eighth grade, however, Nancy and I began losing touch and rarely did anything together.

On a Sunday afternoon in April 1982, I went to Nancy's house. We sat on her front step and just talked, like we did so many times when we were children. Finally, I asked her something that had been consuming my many thoughts for what seemed to be my entire life. "If you wanted to kill yourself," I began, "how would you do it?"

Nancy knew me as well as anybody and was accustomed to my bizarre topics of conversation. Without missing a beat, she said that she would step in front of a train. I grimaced and said that was too messy and painful. Taking my leave from my pseudo-sister, I resumed my wandering around the neighborhood.

I found myself walking down Main Street. At that time there was a Walgreen's on the corner. Almost as if drawn by some unseen force, I walked in and found myself standing in the medication aisle. I looked at the sleeping pills. Taking great care to read the warning labels, I selected a bottle that said that you should not take it if you have asthma, which I had. Quite calmly, I put the sleeping pills under my shirt and walked out of the store.

That night, I took a can of beer from the bottom shelf of our refrigerator. I removed it from the very back so that my father wouldn't notice that one was missing. Before I went to bed, I opened the bottle of sleeping pills, took out the cotton ball, and dumped the capsules on my pillow. I then began swallowing them by the handful.

The beer tasted horrible. My father used to buy this awful generic beer. The neighbors made fun of him endlessly about it, but he didn't seem to mind. The price was right.

I choked down a few handfuls of sleeping pills with the beer, but then had to stop. The taste of the beer was something that I just could not tolerate. I consumed about half of the bottle of sleeping pills with water and then went to sleep.

When I woke up the next morning, I was very disappointed. I trudged to the bus stop and went about my day, sitting in the back of my classes, trying not to do something stupid or draw attention to myself. A few days later, I tried again. This time I decided to asphyxiate myself.

When the weather was nice, my mother walked to work (she had taken a job when I entered elementary school). After she had gone, I took the keys to the family station wagon and went to the garage. The garage door was old and heavy. Its rusty springs and pulleys made a horrendous squealing noise as I pulled it open. Closing it behind me took some work. I had to get on my knees and yank as hard as I could.

Once inside with the door closed, I got into the car and put the key in the ignition. I had never started a car before, but it was surprisingly easy. I sat in the car with the engine running and waited.

I found it very hard to remain seated. I grew impatient. The garage could fit two cars and had a sizable loft. I realized that it would take forever to fill up with the deadly gas, so I got out of the car and knelt by the exhaust pipe. Sticking my head in the cloud that puffed from the car, I tried to inhale deeply.

I coughed. The exhaust got in my mouth and eyes, making them water. I can sometimes still taste it, especially in dreams. It had a kind of bitter taste, almost like dirt and smoke from a campfire. After several deep breaths, I gave up. This wasn't going to work either.

I know that this sounds a bit odd, but I always have to laugh when I think about the next few events. I got off the ground by the exhaust pipe and went back into the car. I turned off the engine and tried taking the key out of the ignition, but it wouldn't budge! I pushed. I pulled. Soon, I started to panic.

I got out of the car and ran to the garage door. It was pulled shut and I couldn't push it open. There was no other way out. I ran back to the car and tried pulling the key out again. It still wouldn't budge. I remember freezing in terror.

For some stupid reason, I was afraid that my parents would find me trapped in the garage and see the keys hanging on the steering column. They would know that I was playing around with the car! The funny thing is that I was willing to let them find my dead carcass, but not the car keys in the ignition! Go figure.

Eventually I realized that there had to be some sort of trigger mechanism that would release the car key. Further, it would probably be on the steering column. I looked and found a little button. I pushed the button and pulled the key. It slid out.

I ran to the garage door and sat on the floor. With my back against the rear bumper of the car, I used my feet to push open the door about a foot or so. With a great deal of squirming, I crawled out of the garage. Standing in his driveway, which was next to ours, was one of our neighbors. He was looking at me like I was an idiot. Taking little heed, I got out of the garage and ran to the bus stop. Again, it is kind of humorous that I was willing to kill myself, but not be late for school. It wasn't until well into the day that I went into a bathroom and found that my face was still covered with soot from the exhaust.

5

HOBBITS, HIGH SCHOOL, AND NEW HOMES

After my two suicide attempts, life got a little bit better for me. My parents didn't get as mad about my poor grades as I thought they would and, eventually, they appeared to forgive me for dropping out of church. Surprisingly, the most significant source of relief came in the form of a book.

In the summer of 1982, I wandered into Beach Grove's public library and checked out a copy of *The Hobbit* by J. R. R. Tolkien. Like so many before me, I quickly fell in love with Tolkien's world of Middle Earth. I read *The Hobbit* and *The Lord of the Rings* over and over again. I must have read them a dozen times that year, if not more.

Much like my admiration of the Beatles and John Lennon, Tolkien seemed to somehow fill a void in my heart. I felt good lying on the sofa reading about hobbits and wizards and rings of power. I loved it so incredibly deeply, I felt that his world existed, that I could somehow go there and be free from all of the misery that I had in the real world. As much as I loved Tolkien then, his true impact on me would not be evident until I was a junior in high school.

My introduction to what high school was going to be like actually began before eighth grade was over. During science class, there was an announcement that all the boys who were going to attend such and such high school should go to one room and all the boys who were going to attend the other high school should go to another room. Slightly puzzled, but happy to get out of science class, I went to the designated room.

There we were greeted by representatives from Beach Grove South High School, the school that I would be attending the following year. It was basically a recruiting mission to get kids involved in various clubs and activities. I really didn't pay much attention since I had no interest in joining anything. I just wanted to be left alone.

Keep in mind that there were probably a hundred other kids in the room. I was sitting in my traditional spot, in the back toward a corner. Suddenly, one of the presenters said, "Would Marc Wolak, Dan Logerado, and Robert Jergen please come see us afterward?"

My heart froze. Anytime somebody wanted to speak with me, especially after class, I was usually in big trouble! Of course, I typically didn't know what I had done wrong. Normally a teacher would point at me and tell me to stay after class. I would then be given a detention slip or a lecture about my "behavior" or "attitude." Sometimes I got all three. I had long ago stopped trying to explain that I didn't know that I had done something wrong. I just took the slip or pretended to listen to the lecture and went on my miserable way.

Reluctantly, Marc, Danny, and I stayed after the presentations were over. Almost instantaneously I was encircled by several of the speakers. Once they found out that I was a Jergen, they began bombarding me all at once.

"Look at those long legs," the track coach said, "I bet that you can run fast like your brother Glenn."

"Never mind his legs," the wrestling coach said, "Look at his arms! They nearly hang to the ground! I bet you can wrestle like your brother!"

I should point out that I was terribly self-conscious about my appearance. I still am. Back in junior high, I was very awkward looking. I literally could touch the tops of my knees without bending! My brother John used to say, "Hey, Rob! Pick up your arms. You are going to trip over them!"

And so it was that I found myself surrounded by a pack of hungry coaches who were all trying to recruit me for their particular sport.

Coaches were to the left of me, coaches were to the right of me—and there was no chance for escape. I only had one recourse if I wanted to survive, and it wasn't pretty. After the initial onslaught had died down a bit, I meekly said, "I have asthma."

There was a slight, uncomfortable silence. Then, in mass, the coaches turned to Danny, who also had an athletic older brother. They started pressuring him to join their respective sports. He looked overwhelmed, almost frightened. But I couldn't save both him and myself. Being left standing all alone, forgotten like a deflated basketball, I did the only sensible thing that I could. I walked slowly back to class.

That was what life at Beach Grove South High was like. I was the "little Jergen." Don't get me wrong. It had its advantages. For example, I frequently had upperclass girls come up to me and ask about my brother Richard, who was a senior when I was a freshman. For some reason, many of my male classmates thought that these girls liked me, a belief that I didn't correct.

Nevertheless, being the "little Jergen" had its drawbacks. For instance, there was the constant comparison to my brothers and the disappointment when I didn't live up to their potential. Much as the coaches left me alone once they learned that I had asthma, many teachers were shocked at my poor academic achievement. Journalism class is probably the most memorable example.

Ever since reading Tolkien for the first time, I have loved writing. I used to write stories in elementary school, but it wasn't until I read *The Hobbit* that I decided I wanted to write for a living. I loved playing with words and creating fantasy worlds. Plus, writing enabled me to be creative without having to interact with people. So, in an effort to prepare myself for my future, I enrolled in a journalism class.

The first assignment involved writing an article on something happening around the school. In all honesty, I didn't work very hard on it. By this point, I never worked very hard at school, as my grades indicated. When I got the paper back, my teacher wrote on the top right-hand corner in red pencil, "C- Your brother Richard could have done better." And so it went.

While my high school teachers were shocked by my poor performance, my parents weren't. By this time, they no longer expected me to do well. During elementary school and junior high, my mother and I would go round and round about grades. I would argue that a C was average and that should be fine. She would say that I could do better if I only tried.

By high school, I think both of my parents realized that things didn't come easy to me. Or perhaps they, like myself, were just tired of fighting about it. Whatever the reason, as long as I passed, very little was said.

In junior high, I was very sullen, dark, and moody. In pictures taken at the time, you can see it in my eyes. There was so much pain and darkness in my heart. I would sit in the back of class and keep my mouth shut as much as possible. Being invisible had its rewards. I also claimed that I was sick at least a couple times a month.

When I was in high school, I became a little happier. I was still morbid and depressed for prolonged periods, but things were getting better. I smiled more and was better able to cope with life's minor adversities. Further, in class, I was becoming less withdrawn and more of a class clown. This, however, would cause its own share of problems.

In elementary school, I was goofy and socially immature. During junior high school, I hid in a shell, praying that nobody would notice me. In high school, my impulsivity became more and more of an issue.

During my freshman year, I was given more detentions than there were days in the semester. Math class was usually where I earned them. I had a teacher, Mr. Thornquist, who was fresh out of college. Every day he and I battled. I did the stupidest things in his class and he would hand me a little yellow piece of paper with the word *detention* on it. Sometimes I would receive two or three at a time.

Once I was called to the front of the class to solve a problem on the board. This was meant to be a punishment for not paying attention. Even though high school was better than junior high, I was still very socially awkward and immensely uncomfortable about being in the spotlight. I went to the board and faced the problem. I had no idea how to solve it and people started to laugh. What happened next was something that seemed to be occurring with more and more regularity. As everybody watched me, I started dancing and making odd noises.

When I present on ADHD at conferences and workshops, I say that kids do such things because, to them, it is better to look funny than stupid. However, truth be told, I didn't think my behavior through that clearly at the time. Actually, I didn't think at all. That was the problem. I found myself in front of everybody acting like an idiot. I didn't choose to act that way. It just happened. It was almost as if I were somebody's puppet or watching somebody else behave like a moron.

I got a detention for my dancing. I also got a detention for writing all over my desk, for throwing paper airplanes, for blurting out answers (most of the time they were wrong and my teachers thought that I was being "disruptive" on purpose, when really I was trying my best), for not turning in homework, for poking the girl who sat next to me, for giggling too much, and for dozens of other bizarre behaviors. I even got a detention for pretending that my desk was a boat. I rowed it out the door and down the hallway. That time, Mr. Thornquist simply closed the door behind me. I am sure that he was happy to be rid of me for one class period.

My impulsivity also affected my grades. As in elementary school, I still made careless mistakes and getting kicked out of class didn't help matters. But it affected my social life far more, especially with girls.

Although I was interested in girls during junior high, I never really tried to approach them. By high school, they were irresistible. Unfortunately, my social skills were underdeveloped and I acted even stupider around women than I did normally. Perhaps the most classic impulsivity story occurred during my freshman year.

Beach Grove South High was a very crowded school. When we climbed up or down the stairs, we were always right on somebody's heels. So if somebody stopped suddenly, people would run into each other's backs.

One day I was trying to get to class, which was on the second floor. As I was slowly making my way up the stairs, I realized that there was this beautiful cheerleader right in front of me. She was barely five feet tall, wearing her varsity cheerleading outfit, and had large breasts—*very* large breasts. Somebody must have called her name because she turned around and, in the process, nearly hit me in the face with her chest. From out of the echoing din of the stairwell, I heard somebody ask, "Are those real?"

Well, to make a long story short, it wasn't until my head was spinning around with snot coming out of my nose, that I realized that *I* had said it. I walked to my next class with a white imprint of a hand on my face. When I got there, everybody could guess what had happened. Even the teacher laughed.

I didn't mean to say anything about her breasts, or about anything else for that matter. Actually, I would never have consciously spoken to her at all. I was an extremely shy freshman and she was this incredibly beautiful upperclassman and friend of my brother. I probably wouldn't have even made eye contact willingly. Yet, for some unimaginable reason, that asinine remark popped out of my mouth. Moreover, I didn't realize that I had said it until *after* she slapped me.

This is an extremely important point to keep in mind. People with ADHD will often say things out loud without thinking. Moreover, we often do not remember saying the things that we said. It is almost as if we are not in control of our own actions. It is almost as if we are not completely sane. You could have hooked me up to a lie detector and asked, "Did you say anything about the cheerleader's breasts?" I would have emphatically said, "No!" and I am willing to bet that I would have passed.

That is how things are for me. I never really know what I will say or do from moment to moment. I have had entire conversations with people and walked away with no memory as to what was said. Even when I teach, I never am completely sure that I covered all of the material that I wanted to cover. It is almost as if I am on automatic pilot. I can guide the plane a little bit, but I can't always steer it to the desired destination. The best that I can hope for is not crashing into the side of a mountain.

People with ADHD also have difficulty regulating their attention. For instance, there are times when I can't read. I can say the words on the page, but I simply cannot put them all together so that they make sense. It isn't that I am unmotivated. My level of motivation doesn't matter. You could offer me a million dollars to read a paragraph and the same results would occur. I simply cannot focus on the words so that they make sense to me.

Reading out loud in school was particularly frustrating for me. I could say the words, but I sounded as if I were retarded, had a speech impairment, or was from a non-English-speaking country. I would read as if there were a period after each word or as if the words were completely foreign.

Even having a coherent conversation is sometimes impossible. I lose track of what has been said or what I want to say. I frequently have to stop and ask what we are talking about or I repeat points that I have already made or I mumble fragments of sentences that seem to have nothing to do with the topic at hand. If a bird flies by a window or somebody else is talking around me, my attention will waft back and forth, never really coming back to what I am saying or what is being said to me. Basically, at times, I am an airhead.

Of course, sometimes I can pay attention to things too much. For instance, I will have thoughts racing through my head and I can't stop paying attention to them. I can't pull my mind away from whatever it locks onto. I become obsessed. It is maddening!

In fact, two days ago, I noticed that my neighbors cut some of my lawn. You see, we have been having an ongoing fight about where the property line is. Several times they have mowed over my flowers and small bushes even though they are clearly on my side. They even started cutting down one of my trees after I told them repeatedly not to touch it.

At any rate, after seeing this small strip of my yard that my unneighborly neighbors had cut, I spent the entire day dwelling on it. I am still dwelling on it. I can't get the image out of my head. It keeps going around and around, getting worse and worse until I can picture them ripping up my flowers, cutting down my trees, and laughing as they throw garbage in my yard. It sounds stupid, I know. After all, they only cut a little bit of my grass, maybe no more than a two- by ten-foot section, but—in my head—it is like they have killed my girlfriend. It gets me so incredibly upset. I simply cannot get the thoughts about the situation out of my mind! I haven't been able to concentrate fully on anything ever since.

I also had problems pulling my attention away from various objects, especially if they are shiny or moving. Just like when my father told me to take the garbage to the front of the house and I couldn't walk away from the television, there are times when I simply cannot take my eyes off things. One such incident still haunts me. It was horrible, almost like watching helplessly as a car is skidding on ice toward a brick wall. To this day, it still gives me nightmares.

It was my senior year. We were doing group presentations in my English class. Much to my surprise and pleasure, I was paired with the most attractive girl in our school. I can't remember her name, but she was beautiful, popular, and smart. She was the "It Girl" of the class of 1986.

When our turn came, we got up in front of class and started presenting the material. As my beautiful partner was talking, my attention was suddenly drawn to a gold crucifix that hung around her neck. I started staring at it. Suddenly, I realized that it looked as if I were leering at her breasts. I quickly turned away. As hard as I tried, my eyes kept being pulled to the shiny gold crucifix. It was horrible! People in the class were starting to laugh and giggle. I looked away over and over again, but my eyes always seemed to end up fixated on her necklace.

After the presentation and class was over, I was walking down the hall. My partner ran up from behind, grabbed my arm, and spun me around. I can't remember what she said, but apparently her friends told her that I was staring at her chest. She was furious. When I tried to explain what had happened, she hit me in the stomach and stormed off, leaving me doubled over with everybody laughing at me.

Another time, I was in a group of students who were being yelled at by a teacher for goofing off during an assembly. The teacher was yelling and yelling and yelling at us. Most of the other kids had the good sense to look at the ground as if they were ashamed of what we had done (I think we were throwing things or talking or something just as evil). I, on the other hand, kept looking around. The more I looked around, the angrier the teacher got. He grabbed me by my shirt and pulled me toward him. Leaning with his face inches away from mine, he said something like, "Are you paying attention to me?" and I said, "Huh? What? What did you say?" The teacher thought that I was making fun of him when actually I simply couldn't pull my eyes off of what was happening around me. There were so many other things happening, I couldn't have paid attention to him even if I had wanted to. Needless to say, I got a week's worth of detentions for that one.

Shortly into my sophomore year, my father announced that we were moving to Indianapolis. He was getting transferred and there was no way for us to stay in Beach Grove. For me, this couldn't have happened at a worse time. I had started to date a girl named Lisa Vorofka and, for a little while, I was fairly happy. Lisa treated me well and she helped me a lot with my schoolwork. Consequently, my grades improved slightly.

We moved to Indianapolis in December of 1984. It was Christmastime and our belongings got snowed in at Chicago along with my first real girlfriend. I started to get depressed again.

The first year at my new school, Perry Meridian High School, sucked. It was very much like junior high. I had no friends. I ate lunch by myself in the corner. And my new teachers seem to have no idea how to handle me. Unlike at Beach Grove South, where I got detention after detention, the faculty at Perry Meridian had a slightly different approach to disciplining unruly students. They spanked them.

Once I got up from my lunch table and accidentally left my tray behind. For some reason, this was a serious offense at my new school. A teacher approached me and told me to report to the vice principal's office. Slightly confused, but willing to obey, I started walking to the front office. But somewhere along the line, I got distracted by something or other. I forgot all about going to the office and instead went to my next class. This, of course, got the teacher from the lunchroom extremely upset. How dare I refuse to do what I was told! I apologized several times and explained that I simply forgot, which he didn't believe. He sentenced me to a week's worth of "lunchroom duty," which meant that I had to walk up and down the lunchroom picking up garbage. I was told that if it happened again, I was going to be spanked!

In addition to school, I also had a lot of vocational problems. During my junior year, I got my first real job at a McDonald's not far from my house. Unlike my teenage coworkers, I actually tried to do my best. But, as with most of my working life, I constantly screwed things up.

For instance, once I was working on the "frontline." Essentially, my job was to call back orders and make sure that we had everything before the customer requested it. It was a very busy day. We had several busloads of kids come in and the lobby was full of people. I couldn't keep up with everything and we ran out of food.

The manager pulled me off the frontline and had me make fries. Before he left he started hollering at me. He said that fries were the number one product that they sold. "We sell fries with everything! Do *not* run out!" he repeated over and over again.

Keep in mind that I wanted to do a good job. Rarely was I willfully disobedient or obnoxious just for the sake of being obnoxious. Again, I really, really, really wanted to be a good kid. So I kept making fries as fast as I could. I had all the fryers working at the same time. As soon as one batch of fries was done, I would put in some more. Fries! Fries! Fries! I made fries like there was no tomorrow!

Then I glanced behind me. There was nobody in the lobby. The rush had passed. I then looked at my station. There were fries everywhere. There were forty or fifty bags of fries stacked in the warming bin. There was literally a pile of fries three feet high waiting to be bagged. And there were several batches of fries still cooking!

My supervisor walked up to me and saw all of the fries that he was going to have to throw away. He was furious. There must have been thirty pounds of fries scattered about. Our eyes met. He was so angry that he couldn't speak. Then I heard myself say, "How is that?" Of course he thought that I cooked too many fries on purpose and he fired me on the spot. It was my sixteenth birthday.

After McDonald's, I began working at Pizza Hut. There I had even more problems. For example, I frequently forgot to put all of the ingredients on the pizzas. A couple times I forgot to put the top layer of cheese on. More than once I forgot the sauce. Much like my elementary teachers reported way back when, I made a lot of careless mistakes, even though I was trying my best.

I also had a lot of social problems. For instance, the workers there liked to play practical jokes on each other. So I came up with something that I thought was really funny.

We had a huge, industrial-sized plunger just in case the drains got clogged. It must have been twelve inches in diameter and sixteen inches deep. I filled the plunger with water and stuck it to the ceiling. A coworker would walk by, pull the plunger, and the water would come pouring down upon his or her face. It was hysterical! At least, it was the first couple dozen times that I did it.

As with my chair-pulling-out joke that I did to Becky Webster in elementary school, I didn't know when to stop. I just kept pulling the same gag until everybody around got sick of it and me. Every day for weeks I would stick the plunger on the ceiling, even after I was told not to. I couldn't help myself.

Another incident at Pizza Hut was far more embarrassing. I am loath to even think about it, let alone put it on paper, but it is very important for you to understand what my life was like. Hopefully, you won't hold these stories against me.

Anyway, I was working at Pizza Hut and I was asked not to come back to work ever again. I guess that I was fired, but I didn't know why. When

I asked, the manager told me that I was "sexually inappropriate" with her. I had no idea what she was talking about. I never touched her or said anything sexual in any way. But apparently this wasn't true.

A couple of days before, I had gone into work to pick up my paycheck. For whatever reason, it wasn't there. So, according to this female manager, I looked at her and said, "Why don't you lay down and pay me that way."

Ugh! I hate even thinking about that story and I am very reluctant to include it here. I don't want people to think that I am a womanizer or anything, but it is an important illustration regarding how little control I had over what I said. Further, many times I was not cognizant of what came out of my mouth. Even comments that shocked other people would not make their way up into my working memory. Unfortunately, the vocational problems that I had in high school would be very similar to those that I would have as an adult, as you will see in later chapters.

Over the years, my life has taken several significant twists and turns. Perhaps the first was when I tried to kill myself. Another was when I was diagnosed with ADHD. Although my diagnosis was still years in the future, something of nearly equal importance occurred in the fall of 1984.

It was my junior year and I was taking driver's education. Driver's education is noteworthy for two reasons. First, as with most teenagers, getting my license meant an increase in independence. Although I really didn't have any friends with whom I could do anything, I looked forward to getting out of the house and just driving. I just wanted to get away.

The second, and far more important, is that through driver's education I met a fellow student named Terry Robbins. Describing Terry is rather problematic. I could tell you all about him, but you probably wouldn't believe me. He was, and is, the most unusual person whom I have ever had the pleasure of meeting. In fact, I remember the first time we ever spoke.

Terry and I were assigned to the same car. It was our first time driving. I was sitting in the backseat trying to wake up (driver's ed was first period). We were going down the road when I looked up. There, peering over the driver's seat in front of me was a slightly crazy-looking smiling face. He stuck out his hand and said rather cheerfully, "Hi! My name is Terry!" Perhaps I should point out that Terry was driving at the time and going fifty miles an hour in the wrong lane while looking backward and trying to shake my hand. That pretty much sums Terry up in a nutshell.

Terry and I hit it off right from the start. He was a nutty and personable guy who always said what was on his mind. He also always seemed really happy. I loved hanging out with him.

Before moving on to Terry's significance in my life, I feel the need to tell you a couple stories from driver's education. I hope, they will delight and entertain you, as well as make you a little more fearful the next time you are on the road. Here we go.

Although he wasn't diagnosed, I am almost positive that Terry also had ADHD. He just screamed of impulsivity, inattention, and hyperactivity! Maybe he should be writing a book like this one.

Once, Terry was driving down a long straightaway. The driver's ed instructor in our car said, "Terry, we are approaching a stale green light. That means that it has been green for a while and it is likely to change before we get to the intersection. So be ready."

Terry acknowledged the instructor, had his hands appropriately at ten and two, and drove carefully toward the intersection at the speed limit, which was forty-five miles per hour. As soon as we reached the edge of the intersection, the light turned yellow. Terry slammed on the brakes and flung the steering wheel to one side. The tires locked and screeched. The car skidded and spun around. Everybody was thrown to one side of the vehicle. When we finally came to rest and we pried our hands off of the door handles, we found ourselves in the middle of the intersection facing the wrong way. Cars were driving around us blaring their horns. Terry looked at the instructor, who was white-faced and breathing very hard. The instructor looked at Terry. Then Terry winked at him and said, "How am I doing?"

Of course, I wasn't any better. I remember a time when I pulled slowly to the line at a red light and brought the car to a nice, easy stop. For whatever reason, the car in the lane next to me ran the light and sped through the intersection. So, without thinking, I went too. Cars from either direction slammed on their brakes and went skidding around us. The instructor braced himself against the dashboard and screamed, "What the hell are you doing?" I had no response other than, "I wasn't thinking." Terry and I didn't pass driver's education.

Back to Terry and my life-altering moment. It was lunchtime and I normally ate by myself in the corner, as I had been doing since elementary school. But then I saw Terry. So, uncharacteristic of me, I asked if I could join him.

Several other kids were eating with him. Terry introduced me to everybody, but they really seemed to pay a lot of attention to each other. Still, it sure beat sitting by myself!

I listened to them as they talked. I really didn't follow what they were discussing, I just wanted to appear interested and social. But then I heard one of them say something about Bree!

Bree is a town in J. R. R. Tolkien's Middle Earth. I had been reading *The Hobbit* and *The Lord of the Rings* nearly nonstop since junior high. My ears quickly perked up. I leaned forward and asked if they were talking about Tolkien. They said that they were and my life suddenly took a huge turn for the better!

As it turned out, the guys who ate lunch with Terry were big Tolkien fans. Further, they played a kind of role-playing game based upon *The Lord of the Rings*. Through Terry, I met four other kids—Doug Uzmad, David Lake, and the brothers Jeff and Dusty Fairhill. For many years, the five us spent our weekends fantasy role-playing. They became my best friends. I am still very close to the Fairhills and e-mail them almost every day.

Role-playing not only gave me something social to do but it also enabled me to be creative and utilize my imagination. The years of developing characters and pretending to take them through dangerous adventures honed my storytelling abilities. It was also one of the first activities that I was actually good at. But most important, it helped me make friends.

Because of our mutual love of Tolkien, the five of us became pretty close. Other than the "Beatles" from elementary school, the Tolkien fans were the first and best group of close friends that I have ever had. They accepted me and willingly interacted with me. They genuinely seemed to like me with my quirky nature and not in spite of it. Because of them, life became far more enjoyable.

6

BOILERMAKERS AND FUZZY NAVELS

Despite my lifelong academic struggles, there was never a question that I would eventually go to college. In fact, the thought of not going to college had never entered my mind, even when my teachers told me that I wasn't "college material." All of the Jergen boys went on to school. It simply was one of those things that my parents expected us to do, so we did it. Several of us even went on past our bachelor's degree. So it is not surprising that, in the fall of 1986, I went to Purdue University to pursue a B.A.

After meeting the other Tolkien fans, high school went pretty well for me. My grades were not very good nor was I very comfortable around other people, but I was certainly happier than I had ever been thus far in my short life. Since Doug was going to be my roommate at college, I expected that things would continue to go well for me and, at first, they did.

I remember the first time that I drove up to Purdue with my father. He was very quiet. Not the disappointed quiet that he was when I dropped out of church, or the quiet that came over him when he was so frustrated with me that he couldn't speak. There was almost a hint of sadness. In fact, as we arrived at Purdue, I thought that his eyes were a little watery. I am not sure if he was proud that I actually got into a college or if he was simply overjoyed to finally get the last kid out of the house. Either way, it was a very touching moment for me. After helping me move my things into my dorm room, he shook my hand, gave me twenty dollars, and left. I was on my own.

I lived at Cary Quadrangle, the largest male residence hall on campus and one of the largest in the country. The rooms were small and the hallways were very noisy, but I loved it from the start. I went down to the dining room and sat by myself at one of the large wooden tables that are still there. After I finished, I leaned back, looked around, and thought to myself how great things had turned out. I was really excited about college and the future.

Oddly enough, at this point in my life, I had two visions of my future. Both weighed equally on my mind, although they were diametrically opposed to each other.

The first vision was what had been haunting my head for as long as I could remember: I would eventually go crazy and end up in a mental institution with a snug-fitting straitjacket holding my arms in a permanent hug. Although things were going better for me socially, I still had a very hard time keeping everything together. My mind still raced with a multitude of thoughts all at the same time. I still said and did things that I couldn't control. I was still painfully aware of how different I was. I would go crazy and I would no longer have to try so hard to exist. As I said earlier, this was a very comforting certainty.

At the same time, I saw myself going into politics. I don't know why. I guess that I just wanted to help people and make the world a better place to live. Even at a very young age, I had very strong, almost rigid, views on various topics. Further, my brother Richard and I used to argue endlessly about foreign policy. Of course, the arguments usually ended with Rich calling me a Communist and me crying in my room. Still, maybe it was just natural that I would give politics a try.

Once, I even wrote a declaration of independence and sent it to then-President Jimmy Carter. I declared that everything within three feet of me was my own country and that I was going to refuse to pay income taxes. I think I was in seventh or eighth grade. I hope that the Secret Service took my letter with a little grain of salt. Many years later, however, I was going to visit the Soviet Union but my visa was inexplicably delayed until after my flight had departed, so maybe they took some notice of me after all.

To prepare for my professional future, I majored in political science and social studies education. However, after taking a few courses, I found that political science bored me. All we did was read about other people's views. I wanted to talk about my own ideas. I wanted to actually do something worth doing. I wanted to change the world! After my first semester, I dropped my political science major and focused on social studies. This would be an important decision because, as I later found out, I love teaching. I can't imagine ever retiring or doing anything different with my life.

Something else happened shortly after my first semester at Purdue: Doug, my friend, roommate, and fellow Tolkien enthusiast, decided to leave the university. At first, I thought that this would be good for me. Doug and I would frequently skip classes to watch the cartoon *GI Joe*. Also, it was clear that we were not as close now as we were in high school. He had several friends at Purdue with whom he hung out and I felt like a bit of an outsider. Plus, he always had girlfriends and I didn't. At that time, I had only dated a couple people and I felt very inferior to Doug (and most males) when it came to my sexual prowess. Unfortunately, as it turned out, Doug's leaving didn't help my grades or my feelings of awkwardness. Actually it had quite the opposite effect.

The second semester at Purdue didn't go very well for me. I was even more socially isolated than I had been before. Further, I had failed Spanish and was put on academic probation.

It is hard to say what caused my failure in Spanish. Yes, I didn't go to class as much as I should have—*GI Joe* conflicted with my class schedule. I also had mononucleosis and was sick for a good three weeks, making me fall far behind the rest of the class. But there was something else that contributed to my problems learning a second language.

As far back as I can remember, I have had difficulty with sounds. Specifically, I had, and still have, problems recalling information that was presented to me orally. For example, to this day, if somebody leaves his or her phone number on my answering machine, I have to play the message over and over again before I can write it down in its entirety. The same is true for people's names. As soon as somebody tells me his name, it dissolves in my head like smoke in the wind. I have always had problems learning without seeing the material in front of me. I also have difficult reproducing sounds. I am simply not very good at it.

Even as far back as elementary school, this problem was evident. Spelling was particularly a problem. The teacher would read the word twice and we were expected to write it down, but I couldn't. I would ask them to repeat the word over and over again. The teachers probably thought that I was being "difficult" or not paying attention, but I just couldn't get the words to sink into my head.

I would also have great difficulty when a series of directions was given orally. For example, if a teacher said, "Take your book out and read pages 132 to 145. Then answer questions 2 through 5 and 7 through 10 by 3:00." I would get everything backward and do the wrong problems. I would probably do questions three through ten and not read the correct pages. My inability to reproduce sounds even led me to receive services from a speech and language person during first and second grades.

In retrospect, I can understand why many teachers didn't think that I paid attention or why they thought that I was trying to upset them. Sometimes I didn't pay attention. This is very true. But even when I tried, it was difficult for me to sit still and focus on what was being said.

My troubles focusing on oral information came to a head in my college Spanish classes. The courses were taught by immersion—that is, the teacher never spoke English. Everything that was said, was said in Spanish. We were expected to catch on by watching her gestures and do what she did.

It was very hard for me to distinguish the subtle differences in the sounds of some Spanish words. To this day, I can't tell the difference between "cerveza" and "cabeza," which mean "beer" and "head." They sound exactly alike to me, much like "pin" and "pen." At any rate, I failed Spanish, and things got worse once Doug left.

My new roommate, Huntley, was from Jamaica. Huntley was very funny. We kept having arguments about whether professional wrestling was real. He said that it was. I insisted that it wasn't. Unfortunately for me, Huntley was also very good-looking and immensely personable with women. He had a new female "friend" every week. As before, I was feeling terribly inadequate as a male. Further, Huntley and I never hung out or did anything together. At least Doug and I had *GI Joe*.

I was beginning to feel depressed and isolated again, very much like during junior high. Further, it was unclear if I would be able to remain in college because of my less-than-stellar grades. While everybody else was partying and having sex, I was sitting in my dorm room by myself, crying. I was miserable.

During my sophomore year, three very important things happened. First, my parents agreed to let me get a single room. I argued that my poor grades were due to the inability to concentrate in the small, confined two-person living quarters into which Huntley and I were crammed. I am sure that they didn't buy that, but my mother was willing to pay half the extra costs for my own room if I paid the rest, which I did.

Second, I decided to get involved. Being social was, and is, very hard for me. I just don't know how to initiate conversations. I have no idea what to say to people. Moreover, I usually say the wrong things and look like a jerk. So the decision to get out of my dorm room and experience life was very daunting for me. After a great deal of hemming and hawing, I joined an environmental group and ran for president of my housing unit.

The environmental group didn't work out too well. The people in it were much older than I was and I didn't seem to connect with them. However, my first venture into politics suited me perfectly!

I can't recollect if I ran against anybody or how many people actually voted for me—but, needless to say, I won. Through college politics, I met my third group of friends—the first being the "Beatles" in elementary school and the second being the Middle Earth role-players in high school.

I can still remember the first time I met my Purdue friends. It was the introductory meeting of all the presidents of Cary Quadrangle's housing units. I had been elected president of "C Unit." I was sitting nervously in the corner, feeling very out of place, when the door flew open and in stepped this odd individual. He had thick, curly black hair, black sunglasses, a cigar tightly clinched in his mouth, a twelve o'clock shadow, and homemade cutoff shorts with string dangling down his hairy legs. As soon as he burst into the room he said in a very loud voice, "Hey, girls, how's it hanging?!" Of course, there were no girls in the room, or I would have been even more nervous than I was.

This unique life-form was Joseph DiGiorgio and he would quickly become one of my best friends. Joe was president of "B Unit" and together, along with a diverse cast of characters, we pulled some of the funniest, although admittedly immature, pranks that Cary Quadrangle had ever experienced. For example, I snuck seventy pounds of marshmallows into a Purdue football game and started a marshmallow fight that lives on in the annals of Purdue folklore to this very day.

Joe was the leader of our little group that we affectionately called the "Purdue All-American Drinking Team." The name was a direct mockery of the "Purdue All-American Marching Band" but it also highlighted the fact that our group was pretty culturally diverse, at least for northern Indiana.

In addition to Joe and myself, the Purdue All-American Drinking Team consisted of Michael Ho, David Dosofski, and Tyler Morrison. A finer group of ne'er-do-wells has never existed. Mike was happy-go-lucky and always beaming with positive energy. Dave was very reserved and thoughtful. Tyler was an intellectual and had a mischievous streak in him. Joe was worldly, outspoken, and very flamboyant. And I was moody and dark. I could be laughing one minute, crying the next, and have a crazed look in my eyes soon after.

The formation of the Purdue All-American Drinking Team was the third important turn of events during my college days. It not only gave me a much-needed social outlet but it introduced me to something that would affect me for the rest of my life—alcohol.

Until my sophomore year in college, I didn't drink that much. In fact, other than my suicide attempt, I didn't drink at all. I was never hip enough to be invited to parties or to get in with the drinking crowd in high school. Moreover, I only went to one party throughout my entire pre-college life and I didn't really want to go. It was right after graduation and there were tons of drugs and beer there. To fit in, I walked around with a can of beer in my hand. I walked from group to group, trying to look like I had friends. Every so often, I would dump the beer out and go get another, just to make it look like I was drinking.

The party was held in a big field hidden behind a barn or warehouse someplace. I was walking around trying to look comfortable when I blurted out, "Is that a police car?" Within minutes, the party was over. Of course, I didn't really see a police car, it was just something that popped out of my mouth! Still, seeing a hundred drunk and stoned recent high school graduates scatter like stumbling rats from a sinking ship was priceless!

Although I didn't drink much before my sophomore year in college, shortly after I met Joe, Mike, Dave, and Tyler, I started drinking voraciously. And it was wonderful! Drinking took the edge off my near-perpetual anxiety. I could relax and not worry about what I said or did. People are far more tolerant of drunks than they are of people with ADHD. If I stared at a girl's chest or blurted out a strange comment, people would chalk it up to the alcohol. Moreover, alcohol calmed my mind down. It didn't race as much. I was less distracted and more comfortable with other people. I could walk right up to a girl, ask her out, and if she laughed at me I could just shrug it off. Chances were good that I wouldn't remember it in the morning anyway.

At the time, beer didn't taste very good to me. So I began drinking mixed drinks and wine coolers. My favorite was fuzzy navels, which was peach schnapps and a little orange juice. I also liked screwdrivers (vodka and orange juice) and rum and Coke.

I drank nearly every day for much of my sophomore year. Sometimes I was with the guys at a party. Sometimes I was alone in my room. Since I was still under twenty-one, I usually had to pay an upperclassman to buy the alcohol for me. For a few extra bucks, they were more than happy to get me anything that I wanted. However, when I went home for the holidays, I was cut off from my regular suppliers, so I stole alcohol from my parents. Once they almost caught me.

My parents had this little liquor cabinet underneath an end table in the living room. Inside, I found a bottle of peach schnapps that had dust on it. I took it and brought it up to my room and, over a couple days, drank it straight.

My parents were never big drinkers. My father would have a beer every now and again, but they never really drank mixed drinks unless they hosted a bridge party or something. For some strange reason, my mother checked on the alcohol shortly after I got home from college. She approached me and asked if I had taken the schnapps, to which I replied, "What is schnapps?" She seemed relieved and let the issue drop.

The involvement of alcohol in my life was fairly short-lived but very important. For the next two years, I drank pretty regularly. The more I drank, the better I did at school. Before I started drinking, I got mostly Cs and the F in Spanish. After I started drinking, I began to get mostly

Bs with an A here or there. I even took the national and Indiana state teaching exams drunk off my butt, and I still did fairly well on them.

Alcohol helped me concentrate. If I had a couple drinks before class, I was able to focus. It also calmed me down so that I could sit still.

Alcohol also helped me socially. Whereas I only went to one party throughout my entire pre-college life, after I started drinking I went to parties every week. I would even crash parties to which I wasn't invited. Alcohol gave me confidence and helped control my near-constant anxieties about being different.

My experiences with alcohol are not uncommon for people with ADHD. Unfortunately, we have highly addictive personalities. Studies have found that as many as 25 percent of children with ADHD become alcoholics, which is *much* higher than the 2 to 5 percent of the regular population. We also tend to abuse legal and illegal drugs.

This is called "self-medicating." Kids with ADHD end up finding ways of coping with their difficulties and alcohol is a very easy way of drowning the feelings of worthlessness that many of us have. Plus, drugs and alcohol often enable us to concentrate better and sit still longer. Don't forget that medications such as Ritalin are very similar in chemistry to street drugs such as cocaine and speed.

Please do not get me wrong. I am not advocating that kids with ADHD should turn to alcohol or drugs. But parents and teachers must realize that drugs and alcohol will probably be a big part of their kids' lives. Think about it this way. If you had a history of breast cancer or diabetes in your family, you would probably talk to your kids about getting regular exams and eating balanced diets. The same should be true for families with children who have ADHD. Kids should be made aware of the potential dangers associated with ADHD, such as depression and alcoholism.

Truth be told, I liked alcohol. I liked it a lot. It made me feel good about myself. It made me feel confident and strong. When I was drinking, my grades went up. I was happier. I was able to concentrate and sit still. The two years that I was drinking were very good ones for me and I still look back on them with a great deal of fondness.

Drinking had a bad side as well. I liked drinking too much. I couldn't just go into a bar with the Purdue All-American Drinking Team and have just one beer. We would polish off pitcher after pitcher. Further, when I wasn't drinking, I had to struggle to control my impulsivity. When I was drinking, I no longer struggled. I just did whatever I wanted, sometimes with dangerous results.

One such time, Joe and I were sitting at a booth consuming enormous quantities of beer. We were both pretty lit up. Suddenly, something hit me in the forehead. I looked down at the table and saw a dart that somebody had thrown from across the bar. The dart had a plastic tip, so I wasn't injured in any way—but I didn't realize this. I flew into an uncontrollable, drunken rage as if my eye had been poked out or something worse. I got up, stormed over to the booth from which the dart came, and started cursing out the group of guys who were sitting there.

Immediately, Joe, who was a kickboxer, got into position should the situation come to blows. Despite my inebriated state, I can still remember the looks on the faces of the guys at the booth. They were terrified—terrified of little Robbie Jergen, the screwup, the kid who used to hide in bathrooms. I couldn't have been more pleased. I loved that feeling. I loved feeling that nobody would dare make fun of me or call me a loser.

As Joe tells the story, even he was a bit scared of me. Apparently, not only was I cursing at these four or five guys (the number grows with each retelling) but I was also saying things about how I was going to rip their throats out of their body and watch them gurgle on their own blood. Again, deep down I have always been pretty grim and angry. Alcohol let lose all that pent-up aggression. The situation ended with the guys apologizing and buying us a pitcher of beer—but the stage was being set for other run-ins.

Sometimes alcohol made me feel calmer and more relaxed; other times it turned me into a whirlwind of potential destruction. I also became extremely impulsive, which was dangerous not only for me but for those in my immediate vicinity.

I remember an occasion when the entire drinking team had gotten together. A girlfriend had just dumped one of us, so there was reason to drink all night. After a pitcher or two, I was running around causing all kinds of chaos. At first, I was just singing "New York, New York" over and over again, but then I started looking for fights. Quickly my friends got me out of the bar and attempted to get me home.

However, home was the last place that I wanted to be—home is where I sat by myself crying. I loved being out with my friends having a good time. It was so exhilarating. So, rather than get in the truck, I ran around climbing trees yelling through the windows of the girls' dorm. All the while, Mike, Joe, Dave, and Tyler tried desperately to keep up.

Eventually, the guys coaxed me back to the parking lot where Tyler had parked. They convinced me that we were going back to my room, hang out, and prank call some of our ex-girlfriends. "It will be a gas," Joe told me. I agreed and let them take me home.

I can still remember the looks in Joe and Dave's eyes as they sat with me in the back of Tyler's pickup truck. I didn't realize it then, but they were frightened and very worried. They later told me that they thought that I was going to jump out of the back while the truck was still moving or that I was going to knock their heads in just for a giggle.

We got out of the truck and I ran to the front door of the residence hall. Joe and Dave were close behind me but Dave was drunk and stumbling around. I turned around, saw that Dave was having problems getting up the stairs, so I grabbed him by the coat and picked him up off the ground. I was intending to bring Dave up the stairs quicker so that he wouldn't keep slowing me down, but Joe thought that I was going to choke him to death. Right away, Joe stepped in and got me to let go.

With Dave sitting on the steps, struggling to get back to his feet, I ran up the five flights of stairs to my room. Joe labored to keep up, but couldn't. When he found me again, I was on the landing to my floor glaring rather menacingly at a freshman who constantly pissed me off. He would make fun of my last name and mocked me whenever he could. I had wanted to beat the crap out of him ever since I met him and now looked like a really good time.

The freshman looked at me and said, "Oh! It looks like Jergen-pergen [his name for me] is sauced!"

I turned around and smiled long and slowly at him. Apparently, he knew that he was in danger because he started backing away. I grabbed him and started pulling him toward the railing overlooking the stairwell, but Joe got in between us and distracted me. When I let go, Joe told the kid, "You better get out of here. He *will* kill you." The word "will" had great emphasis on it. Appearing very startled and more than a little frightened, the freshman left.

After the kid had gone, Joe got me to my dorm room. He then stood outside my door and made sure that I didn't leave. He was very concerned about me, but also concerned about anybody who would get in my way that night.

I don't know if I would have killed the freshman, but I would have taken great pleasure throwing him off the landing. The point is, my drinking was starting to become a problem. I loved drinking. It did wonders for my self-esteem and my academic abilities, but I wasn't able to control my impulses when I drank a lot and I couldn't stop with just a beer or two.

The next morning, I woke up with a sizable hangover. There was a little mirror attached to my closet door. As I walked by it to go to the bathroom, I saw my reflection. I know that it sounds like something from a bad movie, but I didn't like what I saw. I looked at myself and remembered how everybody responded to me the night before. I liked the feeling that people weren't making fun of me. Being feared was much better than being ridiculed. But I also knew that I could have really hurt somebody. I haven't gotten drunk since.

Although my college career certainly was fun, at least while I was drinking and hanging around with the Purdue All-American Drinking Team, not everything was perfect. Classes were going well enough, but not great. By my senior year, I was getting mainly Bs and some As. I did much better in classes that met for one hour, three times a week, than I did in classes that met once a week for three hours. I also did better in smaller, lab-type classes compared to large lectures.

This makes sense. Just like when I was an infant, I couldn't sit still for long when I was in college. Further, I had significant problems listening to professors lecture, especially in history classes where names and dates were thrown about like confetti. My difficulties were so severe that I had to take Spanish seven times before I passed the three classes that I needed to graduate. While I wasn't a stellar student, academics were the least of my problems.

As with junior high and high school, I continued to have a lot of trouble with women. However, unlike junior high and high school, once I was introduced to alcohol, I began dating a lot. In fact, during my junior year at Purdue, I went out with something like twenty-seven women. Unfortunately, I rarely got past the first date.

Dating continues to be problematic for me. When dating, you have to be different than who you actually are. You have to mind your manners and pretend to care about what the other person is saying. There are also all kinds of unwritten rules, such as not talking about past girl-friends, not calling too frequently or right after the date, and not flirting with the person too much or too little. Not to mention being honest! I have gotten into more trouble by being honest than you can imagine.

"Do you think she is attractive?" my date would ask, pointing to an-other woman.

"Yes!" I would reply eagerly.

Needless to say, my date wouldn't be very happy with me. I was sup-posed to say, "No!" or "Not compared to you, sweetie." But I didn't realize this. And even if I did, I still would have been brutally honest. Not because I don't think people should lie, but because I normally said whatever came to mind and the truth was usually the first thing out of my mouth.

Because I tend to say whatever I think, not to mention that I have dif-ficulty picking up on subtle nonverbal clues, dating has always been a disaster. If I really like somebody, I show it too much. I will compliment her over and over again, often to the point of making the other person feel uncomfortable. If I don't like her, I can't fake that I do. I simply can-not maintain eye contact and nod my head as if I am listening like non-ADHD people do. Further, I also tend to forget what I have already said. So I will ask my date the same question or repeat the same boring story incessantly. Perhaps my chief shortcoming is that I can't make small talk. I can't talk about nothing and keep the conversation going. If somebody says, "Nice weather," I will say, "Yup!" and walk away.

At first, I was very pleased with the increased social activity that alco-hol fostered. But increasing my contact with women merely increased the number of rejections and strange looks that I got. I had such a bad time dating that I actually put a list on my wall of all the women who dumped me. Eventually, the numerous rejections and swelling number of inductees to the "Bitch Hall of Fame" began taking their toll. I started drinking even more.

Once, I went out with a very attractive woman and I thought things were going fine. But then she wanted to "talk." As socially inept as I was, I knew exactly what that meant. I had experienced "the talk" many, many times before.

I went to her apartment and she told me that she couldn't see me anymore. She assured me that she really liked me, but that I reminded her of one of her ex-boyfriends and that she often found herself think-ing of him when we were together. She told me that it wasn't fair to me, so we had to stop going out.

By then I was pretty used to getting dumped. I was just happy that I could talk to women now. So I took the "my ex-boyfriend reminds me of you" line pretty well. I got together with the Purdue All-American Drinking Team and watered my thirsty sorrows.

A week or so later, I met somebody else. We went out a couple of times and, again, I thought that things were going really well. But then we had the "talk." As did the woman before, she explained that she re-ally liked me, but that she couldn't see me anymore. When I asked why, she started telling me that I looked like her ex-fiancé and she wasn't be-ing fair to me.

I just started laughing. Granted, I was probably drunk at the time. Still, I found the whole situation very funny. I wondered whether there were a lot of guys who looked like me or whether there was a list of new ways to break up with guys written on the wall in a woman's bathroom somewhere. Joe suggested that there was a secret organization on cam-pus called "W.A.R."—Women Against Rob.

Unfortunately, I couldn't always laugh off the rejections. Woman af-ter woman discarded me after relatively short periods of dating. And there was only one common denominator—me. There was something wrong with me. I was to blame, not the women. To cheer me up, my friends took me to a frat party.

Almost immediately, I met somebody. It was like in the movies. We were across the room from each other with a dancing throng of drunken students in between us. Our eyes met. She smiled. I smiled. Soon, we found ourselves sitting on a sofa in a quieter part of the house. She laughed at my jokes. She seemed interested in me. I was trying really hard not to say or do anything odd. Things were going so well! I was just about to ask her back to my room.

Then she looked at me and shook her head, very much like my teach-ers used to do in elementary school. "You know," she said in a slightly too serious tone, "there is something about you." She paused. Most peo-ple would see this as a beginning of a compliment, but I had more than enough experience to see what was coming next. "You are not like every-body else. You are so . . . different."

I was crushed. I knew exactly how she meant it. Not "Hey, every other guy is a jerk and you aren't" or "You are so refreshingly honest and I really like that." She meant, as so many others have, "You are kind of weird. What is wrong with you?"

After she left me alone sitting on the sofa, I stumbled home and cried. It was 2:00 or 3:00 in the morning, but that didn't stop me from calling one of my friends.

I woke her up and asked, as I bawled my eyes out, "Is there something different about me?"

Being less than half awake, she replied, "Yes! Rob, you are the oddest, most eccentric person I know." I would have killed myself that night, but I think I passed out on the bed. A couple of months later, I stopped drinking completely.

7

REBECCA AND THE ADULT WORLD

The ending of my undergraduate career at Purdue was bitter, sweet, and sad. During my last semester I had to student teach. That was the bitter part. Student teaching was horrible. I admit it. I was the worst teacher there has ever been! I was unorganized, couldn't present information coherently, and wasn't consistent in how I dealt with the students' behaviors. I frequently lost my lesson plans as well as my students' assignments. My students took advantage of me. Other teachers played jokes on me and told my students to "give me a hard time." Things were so bad that I literally had nightmares about student teaching for about two years after the fact.

Also, with the completion of my bachelor's degree, the Purdue All-American Drinking Team disbanded. That was the sad part. We all went our separate ways. Although we still hear from each other every now and again, we aren't nearly as close as we once were. There is the occasional wedding, get-together, or group e-mail, but those have become more and more infrequent as the years slip by.

The sweet part of the end of college, oddly enough, came in the form of a woman named Rebecca. Rebecca was a friend of Joe's girlfriend. During my student teaching, Joe called me one night and invited me out to the bars. By this time, I had stopped drinking, but I still went out with the team. On this particular night, I was swamped with work. I had tons of papers to grade and lesson plans to write. I really didn't want to go out with Joe. I was simply too busy. But instead of saying "no," as I had intended, my mouth said "all right." Now obligated to at least make a guest appearance and then leave, I went to meet Joe at his favorite hang out.

You couldn't have fabricated a better night. It was cold out, being November in Indiana, but the sky was very clear and starry. We also had the bar to ourselves.

I met Joe and found that his girlfriend had brought two friends of her own—one guy, one girl. I am always a bit uncomfortable around people whom I don't know, but they were at one end of the table while Joe and I were at the other, so our interactions were kept to a minimum. I fumbled awkwardly with the introductory hellos, noticed that the girl was cute, and then began talking with Joe.

Shortly after I arrived, Joe spilled a pitcher of beer on his girlfriend. They left saying that they would be back as soon as she changed. Unfortunately, this meant that I was alone with the two strangers. I smiled at them and nodded aimlessly, trying to pretend that I was involved in their conversation, all the while praying that Joe would return quickly.

After many agonizing minutes had crawled by, the guy got up and announced that he was going to call his girlfriend. This was surprising to me, since I had naturally assumed that he and the girl were a couple. Now I was left sitting at a fairly big table alone with somebody I didn't know. She was at one end, I was at the other.

Rebecca and I stared politely at each other. I wanted to say something, something clever and catchy, something that would make her be interested in me, or at least break the silence. I kept opening and closing my mouth, but nothing came out. Finally, I heard myself say, "Nice hair."

"Thanks," she said, "It isn't mine."

I loved that response. It was completely unexpected and delightful. Moreover, it was exactly like something that I would have said. Of course, what she meant was that she dyed her hair and that its beautiful reddish color wasn't natural. But I knew exactly what she was trying to say.

For the next hour or so, Rebecca and I chatted. Joe and his girlfriend took their time getting back and the guy Rebecca came with disappeared, or at least I didn't notice him again. She and I talked the night away.

When Joe finally came back, he suggested that we all go for a walk. Like I said, it was a clear and starry night so everybody agreed. The sidewalks were narrow so Joe and his girlfriend walked up ahead and Rebecca and I walked behind. As we walked and talked, my hand brushed up against Rebecca's. It was quite unintentional, at least on my part, but Rebecca took my hand and held it for the remainder of our walk. It was a very special night and I still smile when I think about it.

I am a big believer in fate. At least, I am now. I believe that many things happen for a reason and that good usually comes out of everything, even though you might not see it initially. When I found out that Rebecca, who was from Ohio, was moving to the Chicago area, I got very excited. When I learned that she had gotten an apartment with some friends in Aurora, Illinois, just a twenty- to thirty-minute drive from Beach Grove, it seemed like we were meant to be together.

My parents had retired when I was a sophomore in college. My mother hated Indianapolis and wanted to move back to Beach Grove. Begrudgingly, my father agreed. So, the fact that I met this gorgeous woman through a string of unlikely chances and that she just happened to be moving near where my parents lived seemed too good to pass up.

Almost immediately, Rebecca and I started dating. Six months later, we moved in together. Six months after that, we became engaged.

I wish that I could say that every day with Rebecca was like that first night. It wasn't. We fought habitually. Further, many of the problems we faced were due largely to my ADHD, although at the time, I didn't know that was what was "wrong" with me.

Perhaps the biggest problem that Rebecca and I had was that we communicated in very different ways. I am extremely forthcoming. If I don't like something, I will say so—even when I don't mean to. If I like something, again, I will say so. As with most people with ADHD, whatever I thought usually popped out of my mouth before I could stop it. I wear my emotions on my sleeve and it is very easy for people to know what I think or feel at any moment in time. As you can imagine, I am a horrible poker player.

Rebecca, on the other hand, was not as overt. She didn't express herself verbally, as I did. She used a lot of subtle behaviors to communicate that she liked something or didn't like something. For example, if she wanted to have sex, she wouldn't tell me. Instead, she would give me a certain "look" that I was supposed to know meant "Let's go to the bedroom." If I didn't pick up on her hint, which was more likely than not, the opportunity was lost.

When she was angry or disappointed, she wouldn't come out and say it. She would become a little quieter and the tone in her voice would change ever so slightly. Further, I was then supposed to guess what was going on and make the appropriate response.

Another source of problems was that I am incredibly insecure. I constantly need to know if I am doing okay and how the relationship is going. With Rebecca, I had no clue. Sometimes she was perfectly happy and I thought that she was mad at me. At other times, she was angry as hell and I thought things were going great between us. I had absolutely no clue where we stood.

This is a common dilemma with people with ADHD. We don't always perceive veiled hints and insinuations. If we are talking to somebody and he is looking at his watch and tapping his foot, we often do not pick up on the fact that he may be bored or have to go. If somebody is smiling at us, we might not be able to tell if she is flirting or just being friendly. There is so much to pay attention to and sometime we miss the important details when interacting with people. As a result, we tend to have poor social skills and our relationships with other people often are strained.

My relationship with Rebecca was pretty characteristic of most of my dating relationships. Although we cared for each other, we communicated and interacted very differently. I also didn't understand non-ADHD people very well, although I didn't realize it at the time.

Frequently, Rebecca and I would sit on the sofa and watch television or read. It was, and still is, very taxing for me to sit for long periods of time, let alone sit in silence. I just feel the overwhelming urge to move around, or—as my father used to say—"make noise for the sake of making noise." So, every few minutes or so, I would turn to Rebecca and ask, "What are you thinking?"

Rebecca would look at me and say, "Nothing." She would then go back to reading or watching television.

The idea of somebody not thinking of anything was incomprehensible to me. It still is. I have always had multiple thoughts ricocheting through my head at any one time. I had never experienced a moment when I wasn't thinking of at least two or three different things. So when Rebecca told me that she wasn't thinking of anything, I naturally assumed that this was her way of telling me that she was upset and it was my job to figure out why.

In an effort to play my part, I would ask Rebecca, "Was it something that I said? Something that I didn't say?"

She would indicate that she wasn't mad.

"Was it something that I did? Or didn't do?" I would press on.

She insisted that she wasn't mad.

"I am really sorry. I won't do it again."

"I am *not* mad," she would say with a stern emphasis on "not." Of course, even I could tell that she was now very angry.

And so it would go. Every week, sometimes a couple times a day, we would have the exact same discussion. She would be quiet. I would ask her what she was thinking. She would reply that she wasn't thinking anything or anything specific, which I didn't understand, so I would bother her until she became angry. I would have the same interactions with other people throughout my entire life.

Another problem that I had with Rebecca, as well as other women in my life, is blurting out inappropriate things at the worst possible times. Once Rebecca went shopping and bought several dresses, which she tried on and showed me. After the third or fourth dress, she asked me the age-old question, "Does this one make me look fat?"

Without thinking, I said, "Not as much as the red one." She didn't speak to me for several days after that.

Another time we had just made love. I was looking down at her. She was looking up at me. We smiled the way couples do. I then heard myself say with a slight shrug, "Not bad." It was just like a scene from the movie *Liar, Liar*! The words just came out of my mouth without me realizing it! She didn't speak to me for a week after that. And it was a lot longer before we had sex again.

In addition to trying to salvage my relationship with Rebecca, I had to worry about working. After I graduated, I tried to become a social studies teacher, but my poor performance during student teaching and the lack of jobs prevented me from acquiring a position. So, in order to pay the rent, I replied to an ad from a private school for children with autism.

Looking back, I suppose that I was always interested in kids with disabilities. When I was in elementary school and junior high, I would hang out with the students in special education, especially during lunch and recess. Perhaps this was because nobody else would interact with me, but perhaps it was because of something else. They didn't make fun of me. I didn't feel like a loser when I was with them. Further, when I was student teaching, I had several special needs students in my social studies classes. I found working with them challenging but rewarding. For whatever reason, fate guided me into special education.

I got the position and began working with adolescents with autism and other disabilities. Specifically, I taught them daily living skills, such as how to ride a public bus or use money. I also got them jobs in the community.

Being in the working world was difficult. At first, dealing with students whose behaviors were as bizarre as mine was the toughest thing. But then I started to get the hang of it. After a while, I really enjoyed what I did. Dealing with people who did not have a disability quickly became the most draining aspect of being a gainfully employed adult.

My primary problem regarding working is not doing the actual job, but getting along with my supervisors and coworkers. It isn't that I have trouble being nice to people. Actually, I consider myself a very good and caring person. It is just that I often say and do stupid things. Consequently, my non-ADHD colleagues don't understand me very well. Then again, I don't understand them at all, so I guess we are even. As you probably can image, I get into trouble a lot.

For example, I have difficulty paying attention during staff meetings. Much like when I was in school, I fidget, look around me, and fail to follow the discussion. More than once, I have been pulled aside after a department meeting and talked to about my "attitude." Apparently, frequently glancing at the clock is seen as being disrespectful. But I can't help it. Few meetings can keep my attention for more than ten or fifteen minutes. Past that, I am staring off into space, bouncing in my chair, rolling my eyes, or sighing melodramatically.

I also got in trouble for saying inappropriate things. Once time, I made a comment about a picture of my coworker's girlfriend. I don't know what I said, but apparently he thought that I was hitting on her. He hated me for the rest of the time I worked there.

Furthermore, there is a lot of paperwork in special education. I detest doing paperwork and avoid it as best as I can. I find it tedious and boring. When I do it, it is usually wrong or I lose it or I turn it in late.

The harder I tried at work, the more people I seemed to offend. Further, the longer that I lived with Rebecca, the worse our relationship got. It deteriorated to the point where she would no longer hold my hand in public or look up from her book when I spoke to her. Finally, I decided that something had to change.

One day I came home from work in a bad mood. A coworker whom I had offended yelled at me all day. So when I got home, I was stomping around the apartment like a spoiled child, hoping that Rebecca would take notice and ask me what was wrong. She didn't. So I decide to go pout in the bedroom, again hoping that she would notice and come comfort me. Which she didn't.

Without thinking, I walked up to her and said, "I think that we should see other people." I was hoping to get a reaction from her. I got a reaction, but not the one I wanted.

Rebecca calmly put a piece of paper in the book that she was reading, pulled off her engagement ring, handed it to me, and said, "Here." She then went back to her book. That, as they say, was that. No big fight. No arguing. No name calling, just a return of the ring and back to reading. If you know of anybody who wants a slightly used quarter-carat diamond ring, give me a call!

With Rebecca and I no longer together and work falling apart, I was a mess. Things were just not going well for me. Once again, my depression was becoming problematic and I was tempted to start drinking again. There were days when I really wanted to stop at a bar and down a pitcher of beer. I could taste it. I wanted it badly, but I didn't have a sip.

As I drove home from work one day, I was getting really upset. I think one of my coworkers yelled at me for something that I did or said. I started crying in the car, making it hard to see the road. Then I heard one of the many voices that bounce around in my head say, "Go back to the last place you felt comfortable."

It sounded like good advice. So the next day I called Purdue University and got information on their master's programs. I moved back to West Lafayette, Indiana, a few weeks later and started an M.S. in vocational special needs education. Soon everything in my life would be completely different!

8

EEG, MRI, A-OK

My return to Purdue University was the worst, yet most crucial, two and a half years of my life. It was far worse than any that I have ever experienced. By the time it was over, the little monster would no longer exist. Somebody else would take his place in the world.

In addition to enrolling in a master's program, I obtained a position coordinating transition services for students with disabilities. As I did when I was with Rebecca, I found high school special education students jobs and helped prepare them for adult life.

While I loved what I did professionally, I was miserable. I was terribly, terribly lonely. None of my friends from my undergraduate days were still at Purdue. Further, shortly after I moved out, Rebecca had a nervous breakdown and was hospitalized for a brief time. For many years, I blamed myself for what had happened to her. Moreover, as the next two and a half years progressed, I thought that I would be sharing a white padded room with her. Things were getting *that* bad.

After leaving Rebecca, my mind was in utter disarray, even more so than usual. I couldn't concentrate. I couldn't think. I couldn't carry on coherent conversations. Plus, the absurd things that I said and did were becoming ever more frequent. People at work hated me and said so to my face.

I can't blame them. After coming back to Purdue, all of the problems that I had as I grew up were being magnified. It was like a fire that was raging out of control. I tried very hard to put it out but the more I waved my arms, the bigger the flames rose. At long last, I was finally going crazy. Perhaps some stories will help you understand how utterly horrible things had gotten.

Shortly after I started my post-Rebecca job, several of the other faculty members took me out to lunch. We went to a buffet where a dozen or so of us sat around a long table. Across from me sat a rather heavyset coworker who had just come back from the buffet line for the third or fourth time. She was lamenting on and on about how she couldn't lose weight.

"I am so fat!" she said repeatedly. "I just don't understand it! I can't lose a single pound."

Then I heard myself say, "Maybe you shouldn't eat so much."

The temperature in the room dropped twenty degrees in a fraction of a second. Realizing what I had said, I looked up. Everybody was glaring at me with not-so-kind eyes. I tried to think of a clever way of turning my comment into some sort of joke or compliment, but all I could do was giggle like a lunatic. Like so many people before them, my coworkers shook their heads and rolled their eyes in disgust.

Shortly after the ill-fated luncheon, my supervisor, Chris, sent me a memo regarding something or another. Apparently, I corrected several of his spelling and grammatical errors and sent it back to him. It was so embarrassing. He actually called me into his office and politely explained that it wasn't appropriate for me to grade his work. I can honestly say that I have no recollection of correcting the memo, or reading it for that matter. I must have done it without thinking—and without remembering it.

To this day, I feel sorry for Chris. Not only did he have to act as a buffer between me and my angry coworkers but he also had to discipline me for the many things that I did wrong. As a result, he was subjected to my bizarre behavior far more than most people.

Chris was a short, happy, former hippy with long hair pulled back into a ponytail. One day, I was walking behind him in the hallway and I noticed that he had a small bald spot. As if I were watching myself from a great distance, I saw my hand reach out and poke the back of his head. I then heard a loud, jovial voice call out, "Bald spot!!!" Regrettably, the voice was mine.

The event was beyond horrifying. It was just like watching the Zapruder film in slow motion. Chris turned around and grabbed the back of his head. I covered my mouth with my hands. He ran into the front office and got a compact mirror from the receptionist. I was attempting to apologize, but the words were falling lifelessly out of my mouth. Chris ran into the bathroom. You might say that he never came out again.

You see, Chris didn't realize that he had a bald spot. Furthermore, his wife had been hiding it from him for years. When I close my eyes, I can still see his expression as he slowly staggered out of the bathroom. His arms were hanging at his side. The compact mirror dangled in his fingers. He had this vacant look on his face. Within six or seven months, he would quit his job, buy a sports car, and divorce his wife.

As I have said before, ADHD doesn't just affect the person who has it. It affects how their classmates learn. It affects how their parents see themselves and how they are viewed by the community. It affects the self-esteem of their lovers and partners.

Like my parents who had to endure the ridicule of our neighbors, my classmates who asked to sit away from me so that they could concentrate, and Rebecca who eventually was put in the psychiatric ward, Chris was just another person trapped in the whirlpool of despair that swirled around me. Because of my stupid behavior, he would never be the same. Further, his children would have to suffer through a rather unpleasant divorce and eventually be abandoned by their father—all because of midlife crisis triggered by my idiotic impetuousness.

Of course, things at school were not going well for me either. My impulsivity was growing on all fronts and people were treating me as if I were mentally retarded. I can't say that I blame them.

During this time, I attended a conference for one of my classes. There were about two to three hundred people in attendance and I was sitting toward the back. The speaker was presenting her research on how children are able to tell stories from perspectives other than their own. To support her hypothesis, she read many stories dictated by little kids. One of the stories went something like this: "I went to go see the Easter bunny. He had no clothes on."

To this I heard myself exclaim, "It must have been a HARE-raising experience!" All two hundred people turned and looked at me. Even though I said such things with increasing regularity, I couldn't believe that I had said it. It was as if an invisible person with my voice was sitting next to me getting me in trouble.

Further, unlike my undergraduate program, all of my graduate courses lasted for three hours at a time and some of my professors didn't give breaks. Trying to sit silently was impossible. I would fidget, look around, exhale loudly, and vibrate in my chair. To prevent causing a disruption, I kept excusing myself from class saying that I had to go to the bathroom. I suspect that my teachers and fellow students must have thought that I had a bladder problem.

As badly as work and school were going, they would soon get worse. Far worse. To this day, I have not experienced a more difficult and personally trying time in my life.

While the graduate courses that I was taking were very interesting to me, they involved a lot of work, especially reading. I would go to my office at 7:30 in the morning, come home around 4:30 in the afternoon, eat, and then rush to class. When I got home at night, I tried to do the assignments right away. But something was going wrong.

For days at a time, I lost the ability to read. I could look at the page and say the words, but I had no idea what they meant. I would read the assignments over and over again. I would even read them out loud, but nothing helped. I tried to do well, but the harder I tried, the more difficult everything got.

I would stay up all night trying to finish my schoolwork, but I simply could not get my mind to function. I could not focus my attention on the page long enough to read a paragraph. Further, I would find myself reading and rereading the same sentence without any understanding of what it was about. Every night I would cry until I couldn't cry any longer. Something was wrong with me and it was getting worse.

At the same time, I was noticing similar problems at work. I have always had difficulties paying attention and sitting still. I have always said and done stupid things. I have always had problems sitting down and focusing my attention long enough to read. But, since coming back to Purdue, my "difficulties" were causing bigger problems than getting mere detentions or spankings. If I lost my job, I wouldn't be able to eat or pay my rent. I simply had to pull my act together—but I couldn't.

Even though I tried very hard to be a productive employee, I frequently found myself staring at the walls in my office or out the window.

I would try forcing myself to be on task, but my mind would drift off and I would stare vacantly into the distance. When I was at my desk, people would walk by my door dragging my attention with them. Several minutes would pass before I realized that I had been staring at the empty hallway.

I also found myself walking around aimlessly, much like when I was in junior high. One moment, I was working at my desk, the next I was walking down the hallway. I had no recollection of getting up. Nor did I know why I was walking around. It was as if my body were under somebody else's control or I was in a trance. Plus, thoughts of killing myself were flooding my brain even more than usual.

More than once, I "woke up" and found myself talking to the secretary. According to her, I hit on her a lot, although I never intended to nor do I remember ever saying anything inappropriate. Sometimes it was like I was on drugs and I just watched myself go through life in a haze.

Things continued to deteriorate. I allegedly called my boss a "power monger." I have no memory of this either. However, I thought that she was a power monger, so I probably did say it. Again, by this time, I was well aware of my inability to remember reality. If somebody indicated that I had said something, I naturally assumed that they would know better than I did.

I got written up for numerous things, including losing paperwork and not getting reports in on time. I also got weekly talking-tos about my attitude and my relationships with my coworkers. While I liked most of the people around me, they didn't like me and they were more than happy to tell me that to my face.

I was about to get fired. I had no friends. I couldn't read. I couldn't think clearly. I cried myself to sleep every night. I knew that I was having a breakdown or that one was close at hand. I would finally get shipped to the white padded room that had been waiting for me all these years. Soon, I wouldn't have to make such an effort to keep everything together. The end was nearing. I just hoped that it would come quickly and be over with.

While all of this was going on, I was working with several students with disabilities. One in particular really frustrated me. His name was Troy.

When Troy was fifteen, he went hunting and shot a deer. As he approached the dying deer, it looked at him and said, "Okay, Troy, now it is time to kill people." Knowing that this was rather odd behavior for a dying deer, he told his parents. Troy was soon diagnosed with schizophrenia and was placed in my program.

Troy's main issue was that he wouldn't take his medications on a consistent basis. He would stop taking them, feel fine for a couple weeks, and then he slowly would start hearing voices again. He got me so angry. Finally, I gave him the best fire-and-brimstone lecture that I could muster.

"Troy," I said not bothering to hide my irritation. "You are such a good kid. You are smart. You are a hard worker. You are motivated. You could do anything in this world that you want to do. Just take your goddamned medication every single goddamned day and the world is yours!"

A little bell went off in my head—literally. It sounded like a little "ding," almost like on a television game show. Then I had this thought that said, "You are such a hypocrite. You are just sitting here waiting for death or the white padded room. Maybe there is some drug that you could take that would make you normal."

The thought that there might be something medically wrong stunned me. It had never occurred to me before that I might actually have some sort of disease or "condition." I always just assumed that I was crazy. The idea of some medical cause of my problems both excited and frightened me. It was a watershed moment in my life, the first of many that would change my world. In fact, to this day I can recall exactly where I was standing at the time. Thinking that I too might be schizophrenic, I made an appointment with my general practitioner.

I remember almost everything about that visit to the doctor. I suspect that I always will. My appointment was at 1:15 P.M. and it was an abnormally cool, cloudy day. I remember approaching the receptionist who sat behind a thick glass window. I also remember that she didn't look very pleasant.

She asked me why I was there. I hesitated for a moment and then leaned toward the small circular vent though which we could talk. Somewhat reluctantly, I said in a soft voice, "I think that there is something wrong with me."

"What?" she asked as if she were annoyed.

I hesitated for a second time and then rattled off the list that I had been preparing in my mind.

"I can't read at times. I find myself staring off into space a lot or walking around aimlessly and I can't remember getting up from my desk. I can't seem to concentrate. My thoughts race round and round in my head. I find myself saying and doing things that feel like they are beyond my control. I . . ."

She interrupted me as if I were a bomb about to go off. In a very slow and overly calming voice she said, "The doctor . . . will be . . . right . . . with you."

I stood blinking at her for a moment and then turned around to go sit in the lobby. There was a woman behind me with a young child. When I turned, we made eye contact. She must have overheard me because the first thing that she did was pull her daughter close and wrap her arms around her, as if I were some sort of deranged serial killer or child molester.

I fought really hard not to cry in the lobby. Fortunately, a nurse soon popped her head around a door and cheerfully called my name. The next thing I knew, I was in a small examination room waiting for the doctor.

When he came in, he sat down and asked what he could do for me. He was rather cheerful, and I wasn't in the mood. I wanted to tell him to ask the fucking receptionist, but I didn't. I took a deep breath and again tried to explain what had been happening to me for so long.

"I can't read at times." I said slowly and began to build up steam. "I can't think. It is like my mind is a pinball machine with five or six balls smashing into each other. I find myself saying and doing things without realizing it. I find myself walking around as if I was waking up from a dream. I stare off into space and can't pull myself back to what I need to be working on. I can't sit still. I can't pay attention. I can't control what I do . . ." I stopped.

At first, the doctor was leaning back with his hands behind his head. After I had revealed a few of my "symptoms," he sat up and took out a pen and paper. For a while he scribbled down what I said, but then he stopped and looked at me. I knew that look. I knew what he was thinking. He was thinking that I was a nut. A hypochondriac.

I started crying. Even now, as I remember that moment, I can feel the tears and the frustration welling up inside of me. I cried, looked at him, and said, "What is wrong with me?"

He paused and it seemed that something had occurred to him.

"You know," he said with a slight nod to himself, "you could be hypo or hyperglycemic."

I had heard of those before! One of my instructors during my undergrad program was hyperglycemic. It involved having too much or too little sugar in the blood, I couldn't remember which. That could be causing all of these problems! I could deal with that! It could be cured! With some medication or change in diet, I would finally be normal!

The doctor ran some tests on my blood. A couple days later, I was back in his office hoping that he had found something wrong.

I sat across from the doctor as he told me that my bloodwork was fine. He then leaned forward, looked me in the eye, and said with a sigh, "I think . . . I think that you have an anxiety disorder." He said this as if it were some kind of sexually transmitted disease and that I should be ashamed of myself.

For some reason, this didn't seem right to me. By that time, I had taken a couple special education classes and we had covered anxiety disorders, so I knew a little bit about them. When I told him that I didn't feel "anxious," just crazy, he explained that my symptoms could have been caused by a slight change in how I was breathing. If I didn't breathe right, he said, the blood-oxygen ratio would get thrown out of whack and I would have problems concentrating and paying attention.

To illustrate his point, he had me breathe very shallowly and at a slightly quicker pace than usual. I got light-headed and felt disoriented. Little spots floated in and out of my field of vision as I felt pinpricks of heat all over my face. My hands felt clammy and I began sweating.

When I told him that this was a very different feeling than what I was talking about, he got a little annoyed. Having a twenty-four-year-old punk with some special education courses under his belt second-guessing his diagnoses did not please him. For whatever reason, however, he referred me to a neurologist.

The neurologist was very patient and kind. I really liked him. He listened and didn't seem to prejudge me. He asked insightful questions and treated me as if I were sane. Further, as a "precautionary measure," he wanted me to have a sleep-deprived EEG and an MRI.

The EEG came first. After staying up all night, I went to the hospital where they made me wear a funny baseball hat with wires sticking out of it. The wires touched my scalp at various points around my head. The technician then turned out the lights and told me to try to fall asleep. I closed my eyes and drifted in and out of consciousness as best as I could.

I had arranged to take the day off of work so that I could get some rest after the test was done. It must have been around 9:30 in the morning when I got home. I opened the door to my apartment, took three or four steps inside, and set my car keys on the kitchen counter to my immediate left. The phone rang.

It was the neurologist. Not his secretary. Not the technician. Not somebody from his office. But the actual neurologist! To this day, I remember the first thing that he said to me.

"How did you get home?" he asked with strange earnestness.

I thought that he was concerned that I drove home after not sleeping for over twenty-four hours. I explained that I lived only about a mile from the hospital and that I got home fine. "Why do you ask?"

I also remember his next statement word for word.

"You can't take baths anymore and you can't drive."

I thought that this was a rather odd thing to say. I would have laughed or made a joke out of it had I not heard the seriousness in his voice.

"What is wrong?" I knew he had something to tell me. Something serious. I also remember his next comment, but nothing else from the remainder of that conversation.

He said, "We found a spike in your frontal lobe."

If this were happening in a movie, there would have been a sudden dramatic sound in the background followed by an extreme close-up of my startled face.

To help you understand my reaction, I think that I should jump back to when I was about three or four years old. It was the first time my parents let my brothers baby-sit me. When they came home, they found a stick jutting out from between my eyes. I still have a scar from the ordeal.

My brothers have never really explained what had happened. Stories vary from year to year. In one version, I was running with the stick in my hands and I fell. In another, I went to pick the stick up and it somehow impaled itself into my head.

The point of this is that I thought the "spike" in my frontal lobe had something to do with this mysterious incident in Jergen history. I thought that my brothers somehow caused all of this. I think that I even muttered "Those bastards!" as the doctor told me what he had found.

What he found is a bit complicated to explain. In fact, the neurologist had to explain it to me several times. Justifiably, I found it difficult to concentrate given that "we found a spike in your frontal lobe" was still echoing in my deformed brain.

EEGs measure brainwave patterns in various parts of your head. From what I gathered from the doctor, and from what I have learned since then, the front part of my brain is far more active than it should be. Rather than a nice, orderly flow of electricity jumping smoothly from one synapse to another, my frontal lobe is like a superhighway with electrical impulses crashing back and forth at the speed of light. It is like a demolition derby when it should be a ballet.

My neurologist didn't know what was causing this "spike" in electrical activity, but he was guessing that I had a form of epilepsy. This explains his first two comments. People with uncontrolled epilepsy are not supposed to drive or take baths because if they have a seizure, they could get into an accident or drown.

The doctor sent the EEG results to an institute at Indiana University that specialized in epilepsy. I was told that they, better than anybody, would be able to figure out what the tests meant. As we waited for their opinion, I took the MRI.

In laypersons' terms, an MRI takes "pictures" of your brain one thin layer at a time. It enables the doctors to look at parts of your body millimeter by millimeter. To do this, they put me on a kind of sled that rolled into a machine where I was supposed to stay very still. As always, this wasn't easy for me, but I did the best that I could. I was afraid that if I moved, I would get zapped with gamma rays and become like the Incredible Hulk.

After the MRI, I went home. This time, I set my keys on the counter and walked around my apartment for a couple minutes before the phone rang. Again, it was the neurologist. This time he was calmer, but something was clearly bothering him. I had just taken the test no more than an hour before. He must have just seen the results and felt the need to call me immediately.

Fortunately, the frontal lobe looked fine. However, it wasn't the frontal lobe that concerned him. It was my brain stem. Apparently, it was misshaped or too big or something. To this day, I can't get anybody to explain it well enough for me to understand. At any rate, my doctor assured me that, while it wasn't normal, it wasn't unheard of either.

What bothered me the most about that conversation was that he couldn't tell me what all of this meant. He couldn't tell me if this was something serious or just peculiar. All that I knew was that there was a spike in my frontal lobe and that there was something structurally abnormal with my brain stem. Although he told me not to worry until he heard back from the specialists at Indiana University, I was terrified.

While all of these medical tests were going on, I started seeing a counselor. Although I didn't believe that I had an anxiety disorder, I realized that I was on the verge of having some sort of psychiatric episode. I was extremely close to crawling under my bed and staying there, much like what Rebecca had done the year before.

Seeing a counselor gave me somebody to talk to about school and work. We also talked a lot about my past and what it was like growing up. I found our weekly appointments comforting and helpful. I highly recommend counseling for everybody, especially kids with special needs.

Also during this time, I was taking several courses from the special education department at Purdue University. One of these courses was on assessment of children with behavior disorders. Dr. Sydney Zen, a very well-known researcher who studied ADHD, taught it.

For one of our assignments, Dr. Zen had us go to a CHADD meeting. CHADD stands for "Children and Adults with Attention Deficit Disorders" and is a support group for people with ADHD. Normally, I would not have gone. Those types of assignments are usually a waste of time. I could have merely claimed that I attended and she wouldn't have known either way. But for some strange reason, I went. Like Chris walking out to the bathroom holding a compact mirror, I left the meeting a changed person. It was the site of my rebirth.

As always, I was sitting in the back of the room, trying to pay attention. After a few minutes, I became really bored and wanted to leave. As I was gathering my belongings and putting on my coat, somebody said, "My mind is like a wall of television sets, each on a different channel . . . and I don't have control of the remote."

I knew exactly what he was saying, so I nodded my head in agreement. A girl from class was sitting next to me. She leaned over and whispered, "What does he mean?"

I explained that he had all of these thoughts in his head and he couldn't control them.

She frowned. "What does he mean though? How can he have more than one thought in his mind at the same time?"

At that very second, my world shook. I could almost feel it. I rarely have moments of extreme clarity. I rarely am able to focus on just one thought in my head, but at that very second I could. It was like the heavens had opened up and the Holy Choir was singing.

I stopped putting on my coat and I turned toward her. In a rather loud and overly excited voice that bothered those around us, I said, "You mean, you don't think of four or five things all at the same time?"

"No!" she said emphatically, "That would drive people crazy!"

"Yes," I said to myself, "yes, it would."

If I ever have the privilege of getting married, if I ever have a child, that moment in the CHADD meeting will still be the third-best moment of my life. It was incredible. One second, I thought that I was a loser. A freak. I thought that I was going crazy and that I should kill myself before it got worse. The next moment, I knew that I had ADHD. More important, I knew that I wasn't alone.

The next day, I rushed to class. I even got there early. Dr. Zen, who also has ADHD, was conversing with another student. I wanted to talk with her and refused to wait.

Butting in the way that people with ADHD tend to do, I started talking, but nothing coherent was coming out of my mouth. I stuttered and stammered. Finally I managed to say, "Dr. Zen! Dr. Zen! I think that I have ADHD!"

I can still picture her turning around and smiling at me. She had this beautiful smile of pleasure and acceptance. "Yes, Rob," she said calmly. "I have been trying to tell you that for the entire semester. You haven't been listening to me. You are the poster boy for ADHD."

I can't describe the weight that lifted off of me. Years of failure. Years of isolation. Years of pain, anger, depression, anxiety, hatred, and frustration were suddenly explained.

I ran from class to my counselor's office, which was also on Purdue's campus. I didn't have an appointment and the receptionist tried stopping me, but I pushed my way past her. Without knocking, I opened my counselor's door.

My counselor was talking into a tape recorder and immediately tried impressing upon me how rudely and inappropriately I was behaving. I didn't care. I stuttered and stammered some more. Finally, tripping over all the things that I wanted to say, I blurted out, "I think that I have ADHD!"

For the second time that day, maybe in my entire life, somebody smiled at me and understood. It felt so good, I began crying yet again. But not the way I normally cried. Not tears of frustration, but of relief and joy.

"I think so, too," she said as she handed me a folder of research articles.

I glanced at them. They were about how doctors were beginning to believe that ADHD was caused by abnormalities in the brain. Specifically, these articles indicated that the frontal lobe and brain stem were probably responsible since the frontal lobe controlled a person's ability to regulate their behaviors and that the brain stem controlled attention. Even though it was extremely improper, I threw my arms around my counselor and cried some more.

To diagnose me officially, I was referred to a specialist who had me sit in a room with a computer. I was told that when an X appeared on the computer screen and was followed by an O, I was to push the spacebar. Pretty easy, I thought. Any monkey could do it.

For twenty minutes, the computer slowly . . . flashed . . . letter . . . after . . . letter . . . after . . . letter. It drove me nuts! At first, I was able to focus on the task at hand. When X and O came in succession, I pushed the spacebar. But soon, I found my attention wandering. I slapped and pinched myself and forced myself to stare at the computer screen. I then found myself glancing around the room, looking at the toys on the floor and the cartoons on the wall.

Suddenly I realize that I wasn't on task anymore. I fixed my eyes on the screen and chanted out loud to myself, "Concentrate! Concentrate! Concentrate! Concentrate! Concentrate!" However, I got so involved in repeating, "Concentrate!" that I forgot about pushing the spacebar. The letters were slowly slipping by.

Finally I decided that I just had to try harder. I willed myself to look at the screen. When X appeared, I hit the spacebar. But the next letter wasn't an O. "Damn it!" I tried harder. Another X appeared. I hit the spacebar. P came next. "Damn it!" And so, with a steady steam of obscenities, my twenty minutes in hell eventually passed. Monkeys, one; the little monster, zero.

The next task was for me to sit with the evaluator and do what she said. For instance, she would say a list of numbers or nonsense words, make me wait a few seconds, and then I was to repeat what she said. She also showed me several pictures of various geometrical shapes, which she would cover up and then make me draw from memory.

All in all, I thought that I did pretty well. I knew that I had trouble toward the end of the computer test, but I thought everything else was fine. A couple weeks later, the evaluator, my counselor, and I met to discuss the results.

There is nothing more humiliating than sitting in a room and having somebody talk about you as if you are not there. Although the meeting with my counselor and evaluator was extremely interesting and instrumental for everything that would happen later in my life, I felt like a little kid listening to his parents and principal talk about him.

The evaluator began by reporting that I stared at her when we first met and said, "I am going to try to act like I don't have ADHD." I have no recollection of ever saying this, but I do remember thinking that the evaluator was attractive, so it doesn't surprise me that I might have looked at her a bit too long. She then went on to say that, during the computer-based test, I constantly looked around and frequently talked to myself, including swearing at the computer. I didn't realize it, but the evaluator was watching me through a small one-way mirror that was partially hidden behind a coat.

She then discussed the purpose of the computer test. She explained that when a person fails to push the spacebar at the appropriate time (i.e., when O follows an X) that measures their inattention. When a person pushed the spacebar at inappropriate times, such as when P followed X, that measured their impulsivity. Apparently, the average person would make about two or three errors during the entire twenty minutes. I made seventeen. Specifically, I missed seven X-O combinations and pushed the spacebar erroneously ten times.

The evaluator went on to say that "the subject had to have the directions repeated three times before he was able to begin." Again, I don't remember ever asking her to repeat the directions. If I didn't know better, I would have sworn that she was making this up.

Finally, the evaluator indicated that I had "significant difficulties recalling auditory stimuli." This was supported by the fact that I could not recall many of the lists that she read to me. My visual and spatial memory, however, were above average.

At the end of the meeting, the evaluator stated her conclusions. First, the "subject" had "severe" ADHD characterized by "significant problems associated with hyperactivity, impulsivity, and inattentiveness." She also determined that I had a learning disability. Specifically, I had an auditory-receptive learning disability that made it difficult for me to process information that I heard. I didn't have a hearing problem. I simply couldn't retain what was said to me.

I remember leaving the meeting and walking around Purdue's campus. I sat down by a fountain and read the report. Everything made sense. This explained all of my problems growing up. I wasn't a loser or an idiot. I wasn't lazy. I didn't have schizophrenia and I wasn't going crazy. I had ADHD.

9

STORMING THE GATES
OF THE IVORY TOWER

Even with the revelation that I wasn't crazy or stupid or lazy or an airhead or any of those things that people have always called me, my life didn't suddenly become perfect. I still had trouble paying attention. I still couldn't sit for more than a few minutes. I still found myself staring off into space or jumping out of my chair and walking around my office as if I were one of Geppetto's puppets. I was about to get fired from work. But, for the first time, I had hope.

After my diagnosis, I no longer gave much consideration to the white padded room. I still got depressed once in a while. I still heard my mother's voice replaying over and over in my head, "Jesus Christ, give me strength! You are such a rotten kid!" I still had a lot of problems associated with ADHD, but I was on a good path. Moreover, I felt that I was finally moving forward.

Shortly following the official diagnosis, I was referred to a psychiatrist. My family has never been one to go to doctors. My mother went twenty-something years without seeing her general practitioner, not even for an annual check-up. I saw doctors, but only for my asthma or when I had mononucleosis. While the idea of seeing a counselor was hard for me to swallow, having somebody find out that I was also seeing a shrink produced a considerable amount of anxiety. For a long time, I refused to go. But eventually I gave in.

The psychiatrist wanted to prescribe medications that he claimed would help me sit still, concentrate, and act "appropriately." But I wasn't too sure. Just as my family doesn't go see doctors, we don't rely on drugs to solve our problems either. I can't recall more than a handful of times when any of my family members took even an aspirin or cold medicine. So the thought taking a magical pill to "cure" my ADHD didn't appeal to me.

From my work with parents of children with ADHD, it seems to me that people hold one of two different mind-sets. The first are those people who stay away from medications, such as Ritalin, at all costs—even to the point of allowing their child to struggle academically and socially. Teachers have particular problems with parents who fall into this group. They get very frustrated and claim that the parents aren't "doing what they can to help their child."

The second group consists of people who are willing to try any pharmaceuticals that they can get their hands on and hope for a quick and simple solution to their child's problems. These people are often seen by society as not "taking responsibility for their kid's behavior." They also are viewed as willing to risk the health of their child for a little peace and quiet.

I fell into the first group. For two or three months, I ignored my psychiatrist's suggestion that I should start taking drugs. I didn't want to rely on happy pills for the rest of my life. I felt that I would be letting myself down somehow if I took them. I thought that I would become one of those people who had to rely on cocaine or speed to get them through the day and downers to help them unwind at night. Plus, I already knew that I had an overfondness for alcohol. So I was a bit afraid that I would become addicted to whatever the doctor gave me.

My concerns about medication are not unfounded. There are serious side effects for any drugs and those for ADHD can be particularly dangerous, especially for young children. In fact, I have heard about cases where children have actually died from various medications for ADHD. Admittedly, these incidents are very rare.

The most common side effects of medications for ADHD involve changes in weight and appetite, irritability, difficulty sleeping, headaches, seizures, and involuntary motor or vocal tics. Recent research has indicated that these side effects are more prevalent than was once thought. Further, there is some question as to whether the damage that medications can inflict is lifelong or temporary. There is significant evidence to suggest that many negative outcomes of ADHD medication, such as damage to the person's liver, kidney, heart, and brain, never go away.

While the merits of medication for ADHD are still hotly debated, there is at least one detail that everybody seems to agree upon. Medications do not teach. Yes, medications for ADHD can help some people sit still and concentrate. However, the pills themselves do not teach a child the skills that he or she is lacking. So if a child is three grade levels behind in reading before she takes the pill, she will still be three grade levels behind after she takes the pill.

Further, there is something called the "rebound effect." Basically, when a child with ADHD is successfully medicated, he can concentrate, sit still, and be in more control of his actions. Initially, everybody is looking at the child and noticing the difference. Teachers and parents praise the child for doing what he is told and everybody is happy. According to research, after about sixty to ninety days, the novelty of proper behavior begins to fade away. People are no longer rewarding the child's good behavior so the child begins to revert back to how he acted before being medicated.

Again, the point is this: medications can help people with ADHD focus their attention and control their behavior, but medications do not teach people how to learn, do math, or act appropriately. If a child has never learned social skills prior to taking medication, he will not suddenly know how to behave after taking the medication. Even the pharmaceutical companies have said that medication for ADHD is most effective when combined with behavioral modification strategies.

At the time that I was diagnosed, I didn't know much about the medications for ADHD. I didn't know about the side effects or the health risks. I didn't see myself as part of any political camp or crusade for or against drugs. I simply didn't like the idea of being a slave to a pill. It went against my upbringing. Further, I was worried that the medications would turn me into a zombie. Although I didn't like much of who I was, I did like the fact that I could be rather quick-witted and very creative at times. I was afraid that medication would take that away from me.

As far as I can recall, there wasn't any one particular event that made me change my mind about taking the medication that my psychiatrist prescribed. I think it was just that things weren't improving for me once I was diagnosed. Yes, I felt more upbeat about myself and I better understood why I acted the way that I did, which was very, very important. But people still hated me at work. I still couldn't concentrate. I still did and said very weird things. I was hoping that the drugs would help me.

For legal reasons, I probably shouldn't mention any drugs by name. However, the process of finding the right drug at a suitable dosage level is crucial to understand. Too often, people are diagnosed with ADHD and they go to their doctor who gives them whatever drug is trendy. The people with ADHD then think that they are going to be "cured" overnight, but that is not how it usually works.

The first drug that the psychiatrist prescribed for me is a very common stimulant. Stimulants have a paradoxical effect on people with ADHD. Whereas they would make "normal" people hyperactive, in the proper dosages stimulants actually calm many people with ADHD down. Note that I said "many," not "all." According to the latest research, about 30 percent of people with ADHD do not respond well to stimulants. As I soon found out, I am one of them.

The initial medication that I took did nothing for me. The psychiatrist played with the dosage level and then tried giving me two different types of stimulants at the same time, but they didn't do a thing either. The next drug we tried hurt my stomach and intestines to such a degree that I thought that I had ruptured something or that an alien was about to spew my guts all over the room. Shortly after starting the new medication, I woke up one night with stabbing pains throughout my midsection. I immediately discontinued taking it—which you should *never* do for reasons that I will discuss later.

The next few stimulants that he gave me worked—that is, they made it easier for me to concentrate and stay seated, but it also made my heart pound frantically and kept me up all night. As I mentioned earlier, these are very common side effects of these particular medications. The doctor thought that my body would adjust and go back to normal, but it didn't. I couldn't sleep and I felt that my heart was going to jump out of my chest.

Eventually, the psychiatrist switched me from stimulants to mood stabilizers and antidepressants. It took about another year, but we finally found something that calmed me down and helped me focus. There were side effects of course, such as slight weight gain and decreased sexual desires, but given that I was pretty thin to begin with and that nobody would date me more than once or twice, the negatives were inconsequential.

The fact that it took me a long time to find a medication that worked is pretty common. It frequently takes up to two years or more before a medication and proper dosage is found. Further, the time can be even longer for young children because their bodies keep changing. Women, in particular, have problems finding effective medications for ADHD because their body's chemistry is thrown out of kilter during their menstrual cycles.

The primary reason for the lengthy time period to find the appropriate medical treatment is that medications for ADHD don't suddenly start working as soon as they are taken. They are not like aspirin. Typically, it takes four to six weeks for drugs to get into the person's system at therapeutic levels. Moreover, if people stop taking a drug cold turkey, they can really damage their body, as I would later find out. So, in order to change medications, people have to gradually wean themselves off the first drug and wait a couple weeks for it to get completely out of their system before trying something new. As a result, the process of finding the right drug and dosage can often take a very long time.

As I was wrestling with the medication issue, I had to also figure out what I wanted to do with my life. My behavior had forever isolated me from my coworkers, and my master's program was just about completed. I met with my advisor who suggested that I go on for a Ph.D. He used to work at the University of Illinois and he knew some people there who had similar research interests as I had.

I remember laughing when he brought up me getting a Ph.D. In my mind, Ph.D.s were really smart, studious people. They sat around dimly lit coffee shops talking about philosophy, smoking pipes, and wearing tweed jackets with patches on the elbows.

While I was doing well enough in my master's program, I was still having difficulty reading and paying attention in class. Further, I didn't think that I would be smart enough to get my doctorate. Still, my advisor made some phone calls and got me an interview.

Much like talking to Troy about taking his medications or going to the CHADD meeting where I realized that I had ADHD, I will always remember my interview at the University of Illinois. I had just purchased (rather impulsively) a car that had a manual transmission, which I didn't know how to drive. I lurched the car around the campus, trying to find the correct building. When I finally got there, I sat in an office waiting for some hotshot professor to come talk with me. Eventually, he showed up.

The hotshot professor was Frank Royce. Frank was, and is, a very big name in special education. He has conducted a tremendous amount of research on individuals with severe disabilities and how to get them gainfully employed, which is what interested me. In fact, he helped create the school-to-work movement that has revolutionized special education. As soon as I met Frank, I liked him.

More than any other teacher in my life, Frank was always very supportive of me and my crazy ideas. He would tell me when something that I did was good and he would tell me when it was crap. But he always stood by me and encouraged me to do whatever tickled my fancy.

Because of Frank and a host of other wonderful people, such as Janis Christensen and Laird Health, my doctoral program was the absolute best time of my life. It was the only time when I could go at my own pace and do the things that I wanted to do. Yes, I still had classes through which I had difficulty sitting and paying attention. But there were so many things going on, it was both chaotic and invigorating. The University of Illinois (U of I) suited me perfectly and I loved nearly every minute of it.

I said "nearly" every minute. As with other places and times, I had my fair share of problems during my doctoral program. However, this time most of my problems did not stem from a lack of social skills, they came from my energy and amount of productivity.

Traditionally, the doctoral program at U of I was a five-year program, sometimes a little shorter, sometimes a lot longer. I was on track for getting done in two years. I was taking more courses than necessary. I was volunteering to work on various research projects. And I was writing my own thoughts and theories.

Unfortunately, a lot of people seemed threatened by my extreme productivity. I dated a fellow doctoral student for a while who told me stories about how our colleagues would complain about me behind my back. Apparently they felt that Frank was giving me too much help while they had to struggle on their own. They also thought that I was an arrogant bastard.

I can understand their perceptions. I got so wrapped up in my exploration of life and school that I wasn't very sensitive to their feelings. For instance, when I finished my preliminary exams, I was surprised that nobody else from my cohort was close to taking them and I made the mistake of telling them that. Understandably, they were extremely offended.

Plus, being twenty-four and the youngest student in the program didn't help matters any. The older students didn't like feeling lazy. They were all very gifted individuals and I made them feel like slackers. Again, I was doing far more than I had to. I wrote my own manuscripts, published articles, and presented at conferences. I even won a national research award.

Of course, my fellow students were not the only ones expressing their disapproval of my newfound excitement for school and learning. There were some professors in the program who found it very difficult to be around me. Some even openly questioned my motivation for working so hard.

Well into my first year, I met with a group of professors who had to approve my plan to graduate early. One of them, an old biddy who had a perpetual scowl on her face, asked, "Do you think that this is some sort of game?" She then chastised me for not "savoring" the program and taking my time to learn from the people who were around me.

This was a load of crap. I was savoring every single minute of it. I was learning more than I had ever learned before. I wasn't rushing through the program to get done. I was eagerly pursuing everything that interested me. It just so happened that I completed all of the requirements long before most people did. For the first time in my life, my hyperactivity, now harnessed and guided, was a tremendous asset.

My doctoral program was the first place where I was able to go as fast as I possibly could and it was exhilarating! I loved it! I started thinking about how ADHD was turning out to be a good thing after all. The question became, not how to "cure" my ADHD, but how to *utilize* it.

I started thinking of ways to increase my abilities. I wanted to learn faster and do things better. I wanted to turn the hyperactivity into a super ability! I wanted to convert my impulsivity into extreme creativity. I no longer wanted to be distracted; I wanted to pay attention to absolutely everything!

I still have the stacks of notebooks in which I brainstormed ideas for improving myself. I sometimes take them out and add new ideas. In chapters 11 through 13 of this book, I outline some of the more effective strategies that have helped me become more focused and productive, as well as much, much happier.

🔟

LIFE AFTER SCHOOL

When I left the University of Illinois, I had just turned twenty-seven. For the first time in my life, I was doing well, more or less, on all fronts. With the exception of two Bs, I had gotten all As in my doctoral program, so I was learning better than ever before. I didn't have many friends, but I was dating somebody on a regular basis. And, most important, I was coming to grips with who I was. I still had very low self-esteem at times, but for the most part, I was happy. The thought of the white padded room was slowly fading from my mind.

As I was finishing up my dissertation, I was offered a job at Southwest Missouri State University (SMSU). Much to my disappointment, leaving the University of Illinois and going to SMSU was like running into a brick wall at full speed.

At Illinois, I had a wonderful mentor who looked out for me, taught me what I needed to know, and increased my confidence. He always gave me opportunities to learn and would praise me up and down when I did good work. He also accepted me for who I was and overlooked my "uniqueness." Without him, I wouldn't have made it through my doctoral program.

At SMSU, people were very different. They were intolerant and expected me to "fit in" the way that they wanted. They also refused to help me in any way. For instance, I was given a small office with pale concrete walls and flickering fluorescent lights. The office didn't have any windows, making me feel like I was in solitary confinement or something.

I explained that I couldn't concentrate in such a setting and asked for a different office, specifically one with a window. My request was denied. I asked that the lights be fixed, but they never got around to it. I offered to paint the walls myself, but I was told that I couldn't. That wasn't allowed.

Finally, I was going to make a formal request for accommodations under the Americans with Disabilities Act, or ADA, but I was told that I was being "demanding." Moreover, senior faculty members not so subtly implied that I needed to learn how to "get along" and "not rock the boat"—that is, if I wanted to become tenured.

As a result of my intolerable office, I started working at home. I would come to school for my office hours and when I had class, but I did all of my writing and grading at my apartment or the library. Apparently, my colleagues thought that I was being standoffish. They complained to my department chair that I wasn't being a "team player," so my department chair required that I be in my office every day, which decreased my productivity tremendously.

Perhaps the biggest problem that I had at SMSU came as the result of my own impulsivity. Specifically, I found out that a colleague was falsifying her research and, without thinking, I confronted her about it. Actually, I wasn't going to say anything to her at all. I was going to discreetly take my evidence through the proper channels and be professional. However, as soon as I saw her, I blurted out something like, "I know that you are cooking your data!" ("Cooking" is a term for rigging the results of a study so it shows something worth publishing.) Immediately things at work got very hostile and, after only two semesters, I decided to leave SMSU.

Fortunately, Ph.D.s in special education are in relatively short supply. Further, coming from the University of Illinois as well as being Frank Royce's student, I was able to get a position at the Institute on Developmental Disabilities in Chicago.

At SMSU, I was expected to teach and do research on the side. At the institute, I did nothing but research. While I enjoy conducting studies, I had a very hard time performing my new job. I was expected to produce on command. Somebody would hand me a stack of articles and I was expected to read them right then and there. I couldn't operate that way. I still can't. Sometimes I can read, sometimes I can't. The people in my new job didn't seem to understand this. I soon found that the institute was the wrong place for me as well.

While at the institute, I realized that I missed teaching. Plus, the eight-to-five-type job didn't suit me. I wanted something with more flexibility. So, if I couldn't focus enough to read or write, I would be allowed to do my work when I could. For the second time in two years, I started applying for positions.

Soon, I got positions at Loyola University and Northern Illinois University. Here, I was given temporary, one-year contracts to teach in their respective special education departments. In both positions, I did fairly well. Being an ad hoc professor made it very easy for me to simply do my job without too much contact with my coworkers. But I needed something more permanent if I was ever going to settle down.

After bouncing around from university to university, I finally came to rest at a university in Wisconsin, which is where I am today. This is the fifth university that I have been at since earning my Ph.D. Although I have stayed here for five years now, it hasn't always gone well for me.

I want to point out that the people at the University of Wisconsin (UW) are, for the most part, very nice. I like many of them, although I am not very close to anybody in particular. They do their thing, and I do mine. As nice as they are, it took me a long time to educate them about ADHD and there are still some people who are reluctant to listen to what I have to say on the topic. Moreover, many of my colleagues simply don't understand me or appreciate my oddities.

For instance, my office is a mess. I mean, it is absolutely filthy. Twice, I have had the fire marshal come and tell me to clear a sixteen-inch-wide path from my desk to the door!

For some reason, people feel the need to come into my office and point out what a slob I am. People I don't even know will poke their heads into my office and make very rude comments. Then, when I get upset, they think that I am being unreasonable. After all, my office *is* messy and they feel that they have a right to point it out to me.

During one of my first days at my new job, I was working at my desk, being productive, when another professor came in and said, "This is a fucking pigsty! If you don't clean it up, at least have the courtesy to close your door." This was good advice. I now keep my office door closed, although some people interpret this as if I am being aloof.

What makes me angry is that people tell me that I have poor social skills, but I have never gone into somebody's house and willingly said, "Geez! Get a maid! You are a P.I.G.—PIG!" Yet, non-ADHD people can get away with being rude. When they do it, it is considered "good-natured teasing." When I do it, I am being "inappropriate."

Another problem that I have had at UW involves how other faculty view ADHD. Specifically, some do not believe that ADHD exists. They feel that it is just a trendy way of shifting the blame for "poor parenting" to the child's brain. Other faculty members say that ADHD is an actual condition, but that I don't have it. More than once I have been told that I couldn't have ADHD because I earned a Ph.D. Apparently, from their viewpoint, people with ADHD are stupid or not able to succeed.

This is probably one of the biggest obstacles that most children with ADHD will have to overcome. Parents and teachers tell children with ADHD that they can't do this or that. They will say, "Oh, you can't sit still because of your ADHD" or "You aren't going to be able to do well in school because of your disability." So the child believes what she is told and then lives up to everybody's low expectations. In other words, she will be limited not by her own abilities but by other people's perceptions. After all, if parents and teachers don't believe that children with ADHD can succeed, the children won't believe it either. And if the children don't think that they can accomplish anything, why should they even try?

My first couple years at UW were challenging primarily because many senior faculty members held this negative view of people with disabilities. Further, my department chair, in particular, couldn't understand what it was like having ADHD. He would barge into my office, demanding to speak with me about something that I had done wrong. I would explain to him that I was busy and that if I got off track, it would be very hard for me to get back on track, but he didn't care. He felt that I should be able to "recover from a minor distraction."

This, of course, simply isn't the case. For people with ADHD, being able to concentrate is a very transitory event. It is like the weather. One minute it is bright and sunny and I can focus my attention with remarkable clarity. The next moment, clouds are rolling in and my head is filled with a fog. Consequently, I take great care to utilize the times when I can think and I do my best not to let them slip away. That is why I do not tolerate interruptions and try to minimize them as much as possible.

Most non-ADHD people can't appreciate this. They think that people can read or write or think whenever they want, so it shouldn't be too hard to take a couple seconds to answer a few questions or say hello. However, in those seconds, I not only lose my train of thought but the entire train disappears along with the tracks.

Something else my department chair and colleagues don't understand is that I am not always conscious of what I say or do. Not only do I forget things but I also have very little comprehension as to what I am saying at any one moment. Later, when I get in trouble and I say, "I don't remember doing that" everybody assumes that I am lying.

For instance, once I was visiting one of my students at the school where she was student teaching. As we were standing in the hallway, reviewing how things were going, a very attractive female teacher who was my age walked by. According to my student, I "leered" at the teacher and then asked my student if the teacher was single. The student filed a complaint saying that I made her feel like my "pimp" and that it wasn't her job to keep track of who was available for dating. (I find it interesting that this complaint came after I wrote a less-than-favorable review of the student and not immediately after the alleged incident had occurred.)

Anyway, when I was called down to the office to discuss this incident, my department chair told me several times that if I just "tried harder" I wouldn't say such inappropriate things. He didn't understand. I *was* trying. I just had a tendency to say things that offended people.

Further, when I told my department chair that I didn't recall making any of these offensive comments, he clearly thought that I wasn't telling the truth. "How can you not remember saying such things?" he said in utter frustration. He didn't get it. There are some things that stick in my head for years, so it isn't like I can't remember anything. But I am never completely aware of what my mouth is saying at any moment in time. It is like I can't distinguish between what I am thinking and what I am saying.

I should point out that my relationship with my department chair is much better now than it once was, especially compared to my first year here. Although I don't think he truly understands me, he has made an effort to tolerate me, which I greatly appreciate. I have also made an effort to have only positive interactions with him. So while my ADHD has caused some rough spots here, most of the spots have been smoothed out.

Another time, I was talking with one of my student teacher's onsite supervisors. She had been ill for a very long time and just come back to work after an extended medical leave. As we chit-chatted, I was about to say, "You look great!" but I realized that that could be considered sexual harassment, so I bit my tongue as best as I could. Suddenly, as she paused in her story about how sick she was, I heard myself say, "But you look great!" I immediately covered my mouth, but it was too late. The comment had already escaped.

I apologized up a storm and explained that I didn't mean anything improper. She just laughed. Fortunately, she understood what I was trying to say and didn't take offense. I wish everybody would be so tolerant of compliments, but they aren't. Most people nowadays seem to get offended about every little comment, especially if it has something even vaguely associated with sex or somebody's appearance.

For this reason, working with some students is very tough for me. Special education is overwhelmingly female. I would guess that about 95 percent of my students are females in their early twenties. Given that I am close to many of their ages and that I say whatever comes into my mind, working with them is particularly anxiety provoking. I am perpetually afraid of saying or doing anything that might be considered sexual harassment. Whenever I blurt out something like "Nice jacket" or "I like your haircut," I immediately say "But I don't mean anything by that." Usually students just laugh, but some have gotten livid.

During my first couple years in Wisconsin, several students lodged complaints against me. One of them was an older student in her fifties. She called me at home to bitch about her grade. When I picked up the phone, she said, "This is so-and-so. I am in your class. Do you know who I am? I sit at the corner table."

I average a hundred students or more a year, so I don't know many of them by name. Nevertheless, I thought that I knew this student; but I wasn't sure. There were, after all, four corner tables in the classroom and all of them had a woman sitting at them. So I asked, "Are you the blonde who sits to the back of the class and to my left?"

All hell broke out. Apparently referring to somebody's hair color can be considered sexually inappropriate. Of course, if the student had been passing my class, I am sure that she wouldn't have complained at all.

At the beginning of my second year here, I formally requested accommodations for my "disability." Specifically, I wanted things presented to me in writing because I had missed a couple of meetings that somebody told me about in passing. As I have said, I simply don't remember auditory information very well. I also wanted students who were complaining to come to me before they filed any complaints with my department chair or the dean. Finally, I wanted a mentor, a tenured faculty member, who would work with me on some of these issues. I needed an advocate like I had during my doctoral program, somebody who would talk to me and help me if I did something wrong.

I met with people from the university and presented my concerns and needs. Unfortunately, as at Southwest Missouri State University, my request for accommodations was denied. I was told that things were going to go fine for me and that I should just wait and see how everything turned out.

Regrettably, even some of the nicer people at UW don't seem to appreciate what it is like to have ADHD. Regularly, as I sit in my office working, people come in and start talking to me. I have tried explaining that it is really hard for me to get back on track once I have been derailed, but they don't understand. Nearly every day it is the same thing. I am working and somebody will come into my office, sit down, and start chit-chatting with me. I know that they are merely being pleasant. They want to socialize and be part of my life, but it is impossible for me to be productive when I keep being interrupted every few minutes.

Not only do my colleagues not understand ADHD, they cannot comprehend why I think it is a gift. Once, a group of us was standing in the front office talking about somebody who was expecting a baby. Somebody said something to the effect of, "I just hope it is happy, healthy, and doesn't have any disabilities." I blurted out, "I hope that it has ADHD!" Immediately one of the people hit me in the shoulder. Not to be a whiner, but it hurt!

Again, if I had hit somebody as result of my impulsivity, I would get in trouble, which I told her, but she just laughed at me. There seems to be this double standard between what people with and without ADHD can do. If a non-ADHD child gets out of his seat during class, the teacher might ask him to sit back down. If a child with ADHD gets out of his seat, the teacher tells the parents to increase the child's medication. So it goes.

Of course, life after my doctoral program hasn't been all work. I have been able to make a few friends here and there. The problem with making friends is that I am not very comfortable around people I don't know. I can't make small talk. I am very direct and to the point. This, as well as the fact that I tend to say bizarre things, limits my opportunities to make lasting friendships. Plus, I tend to move from job to job a lot, so I don't get to be around people for an extended period.

Dating is particularly problematic, as I mentioned in previous chapters. There are all kinds of subtle rules to dating that I have great difficulty following. You are not supposed to call the other person too soon or too often. You can't be too open right away—et cetera, et cetera, et cetera.

Once, when I was in Missouri, I had gone out with somebody a couple times. I really liked her. Unfortunately, I "accidentally" called her three or four times in one day. I didn't mean to be a pest or look desperate; I just forgot that I had already called her earlier in the day. It was as if every time I thought about her, I started dialing the phone before I realized that I had already left a couple messages.

Another problem that I have with dating is getting past the first date. People with ADHD, including myself, not only have problems understanding the rules that we are supposed to adhere to but we also have difficulty being anyone other that who we are. I simply can't "act normal." For instance, I once went to a woman's house to pick her up for our first date. As she was getting ready, I was sitting in her living room looking through her video collection. Apparently, she asked me what I was doing and I replied, "Looking for porn." Of course, I don't remember saying this at all and I was probably just joking. But the point is, I really liked the girl and was trying to be on my best behavior. Yet, even on my best behavior, I say stupid things.

Another time, my date and I were talking in her kitchen. As she was telling me a story, I felt a hair in my mouth so, without thinking, I pulled the hair out and wiped it on her sweater! She stopped telling her story, looked at the slobbery hair, looked at me, and then said, "You realize that I saw you do that, don't you?" Why she put up with me, I will never know.

Perhaps the worst aspect of dating for me is paying attention to what is being said. I simply do not have the capacity to sit smiling at somebody, nodding my head, and saying the traditional "Ah ha" at the appropriate times. When I am bored, my face shows it immediately.

Even when I am very interested in the conversation, it is very hard for me to maintain eye contact, especially when a lot is happening around us. My eyes constantly go this way and that, following the slightest movement. On several different occasions, outings have ended early because my dates thought that I was looking at other women. Even my female friends have pointed out that I look at women a lot.

I believe that this is unfair. It isn't that I "look" at other women; I simply glance at anybody or anything that moves around me. My female friends and dates only notice when it is a woman who catches my eye. They don't say a thing when I get distracted by a guy or a bird flying past the window.

One time, I was sitting at a restaurant, talking with somebody whom I had just met. I thought that things were going pretty well. I was interested in her and she seemed interested in me. Suddenly, she throws her napkin at my face and says, "Go ahead and ask her out, too!"

Of course I had no idea what she was talking about and told her so in probably those exact words. She said that I had been ogling a busty waitress throughout the entire evening and that I was an asshole. She then got up and stormed out of the restaurant. I never heard from her again.

Yes, there are times when I can't take my eyes off of people, especially if they are really attractive or odd looking. Many times I have found myself staring at pretty women or guys with bad toupees or gunk in their teeth or whatever. However, more often than not, I simply glance around and do not even realize what I am seeing. In fact, I didn't even realize that the waitress was busty until my date had pointed it out to me.

My friends are very aware of this behavior and tolerate it with remarkable goodwill. One of them likens it to me watching a butterfly. She says my gaze floats around from here to there, never really coming to rest on anything in particular for very long. She thinks it is funny, but my inability to focus my attention is very problematic in numerous areas of adult life, such as interviewing for jobs.

I have interviewed for many, many jobs. On paper, I am told that I look pretty impressive. I have numerous publications and have presented all over the country. Plus, I came from very good universities and have great teaching evaluations.

Although I am likely to get an interview for the majority of positions for which I apply, I rarely get offered the appointment. As a matter of fact, I have gone into interviews being told that it was "just a formality" and that the job was mine if I wanted it, only to get a form letter a few weeks later saying that somebody else had been hired.

As with dating, interviews have unwritten rules and expectations. For example, while it is considered good form to make small talk about items that interviewers have in their offices, it is not appropriate to look at pictures of their teenage daughters and say, "Wow! She's a *babe!*"—which I have done twice!

Further, interviews for faculty positions tend to last all day for a couple days straight. Just as I have trouble paying attention during an hour dinner with a date, I simply cannot force myself to pay attention during ten- to twelve-hour-long interviews. By the second or third hour, I usually give up trying and merely hope for the best.

Furthermore, I tend to do and say things that are completely tactless. For instance, I interviewed in Hawaii a couple of years ago. As I got off the plane, the faculty member who was picking me up from the airport put a lei around my neck and went to kiss my cheek, as is the custom there. Without thinking, I turned my head and kissed the woman full on the lips with a little too much enthusiasm. Needless to say, I didn't get that job.

During another occasion at a different university, the entire faculty was interviewing me at the same time. They were introducing themselves and asking me various questions. A very old and well-respected professor pointed out that he went to Indiana University for his doctorate, to which I replied, "I'll try to use smaller words for you." There was a dead silence and he never finished his point.

Although there is good-natured ribbing between Purdue graduates, such as myself, and people from Indiana University, such polite teasing isn't appropriate on a job interview. I wasn't offered that position either!

A part of nearly every interview is "the meal." Usually faculty members take candidates out to eat at fancy restaurants in order to impress them. During a particular interview, I was invited to a faculty member's home where I met his family. As we were eating, his wife asked me what I thought of the dinner, which she had obviously cooked. Without looking up from my plate and my mouth partly full of food, I heard myself say, "It is a bit dry." There was an awkward pause and then I heard myself add, "and it needs more salt or something to give it taste." I didn't get that job either.

Unfortunately, my poor interviewing skills conflict greatly with my desire to relocate every year or so. Frequently, I have an overwhelming urge to change jobs and move. I get bored with my surroundings and want something new and exciting. As an impulse, I will send out résumés to anybody who has a position that even remotely matches my qualifications.

This is pretty typical of adults with ADHD. Whereas children with ADHD are overtly physically hyperactive, adults with ADHD tend to experience periods of extreme restlessness. It becomes a kind of compulsion. We have to move and try something new. Boredom is hell for people with ADHD. One way to combat this boredom is to move from job to job and place to place. We often leave our jobs and homes without much thought or planning. Several of my ADHD acquaintances have quit their jobs before they have secured new ones or put their homes up for sale without any idea where they were going to live once it sold.

Though I haven't been as rash as some people, I check the professional journals for position openings every day. I am never completely happy or settled wherever I am. I always seem to think that another town or another job will hold my attention better than the one that I am in. The running joke among my friends is that I can be "unhappy anywhere."

When I took my current job, I knew that I would want to leave after a few months, so I bought a house to help anchor me down. While I still have the desire to move, having a house that I would have to sell prevents me from packing up and leaving whenever the mood hits me. Of course, having a house also has presented me with many interesting challenges.

For example, like my office, my homes have always been very messy, particularly my bedrooms and kitchens. They are so messy that I am very embarrassed to have people over. Thankfully, my poor social skills and lack of friends keep visitors to a minimum.

In addition to being messy, I tend to start a lot of projects around the house, but few of them ever seem to get completed. For instance, I began painting the outside of my house two years ago. Two of the sides are finished; the two others remain half painted.

Further, I love gardening. I find it very relaxing, yet physically demanding. So every spring, I dig up large parts of my yard and plant various seeds and bulbs. However, I never have the patience to water them. Consequently, I have many patches of dirt and weeds growing here and there around my house.

My lawn is not the only thing to suffer from my impulsivity. Without thinking, I decided to trim the cords that hang from my window blinds. So I went around the house with scissors trimming the unsightly cords that hung down. I even tried to make sure that all of the cords were the same length. Again, I usually mean well, I just have a tendency of screwing things up.

Halfway through the trimming, I realized that if I cut the cords, I couldn't lower the blinds. Now half of my window blinds cannot be lowered more than a few inches.

My distractibility has also caused many problems too. I love the smell of scented candles. They help me unwind. Plus, they make the house smell good. Unfortunately, I frequently leave candles burning unattended. I live in constant fear of burning my house down.

Moreover, I often leave the stove and oven on, sometimes for days at a time. I burn food. I forget to put food back in the refrigerator and it spoils. I forget about my dinner and leave it where my cats can get to it. I try to cook something nice, but forget to put in key ingredients, such as butter or sugar. So it goes.

Once I was cooking chicken wings. I put them on a cookie sheet in the oven. When they were just about done, I turned off the oven and basted the wings with a final coat of sauce. To make a long story short, I found the blackened remains of the wings a couple of weeks later. Oddly enough, they tasted fine.

Perhaps the most potentially detrimental problem that I have is paying my bills on time. I make a concerted effort to pay them as soon as they arrive, but I nearly always forget. Further, I habitually lose them or put them in places where I can't find them when I need them, such as my coat or pants pocket. Moreover, when I do remember to pay my bills, I repeatedly forget to put stamps on the envelopes. I have even forgotten to put the checks with the statements. Luckily, I now have most of my bills directly paid by the bank, which helps a great deal.

Despite all of the difficulties that I have had, despite the anxiety, the social and academic failures, the loneliness, the depression . . . despite everything that I have been telling you, life has turned out amazingly well. I am now glad that I have ADHD. In fact, as I said in the opening of this book, I wouldn't want to be any other way. I have ADHD and that is A-OK!

A LOOK AT THE PRESENT

As I have said, my life is going pretty well, despite how things began. I was recently given tenure and promoted to associate professor. I have written over thirty articles and seven books during the past five years. I have presented papers all over the country about ADHD and have been interviewed by *USA Today*, *Time*, and *Working Woman* magazines regarding my view that ADHD is a gift. I live comfortably in a beautiful, albeit messy and half-painted, house. I even have a wonderful girlfriend whom I love dearly and have been dating for over two years. I hate to say it because it sounds so egotistical, but I guess that I am a "success."

I still have problems at work now and again, especially with saying things without thinking. For instance, during my last departmental meeting, we gave a colleague who was moving away a gift certificate for Home Depot. The colleague said, "Whatever I buy, I will always think of all of you when I look at it." I blurted out, "I hope you don't get a toilet!" Thankfully, people laughed.

Of late, I have been getting along better with my colleagues and students. Now that my students know that I have ADHD, they are far more tolerant of my behavior. At least most of them are. This semester, a couple of students actually tried to use my ADHD against me!

The two students in question turned in nearly identical final projects for my class. When I confronted them about it, they tried convincing me that I had said that it was okay to work together. One of them even went so far as to say, "Oh, you must have forgotten that you said that because of your ADHD." I know damn well that I didn't say that they could work together. They just wanted to cheat. Fortunately, I had several honest students from the class come forward and tell me that I never said anything about collaborating. As you can imagine, it is a constant struggle to keep track of what I say, to whom, and when. Writing things down immediately helps tremendously.

I had another student this semester who wrote a letter to the dean complaining that I refused to read over her assignment and explain why she missed points. I didn't refuse to help her. I simply said that I couldn't read it right then and there because I was too hyper and distractible. She didn't understand and left the room in a big huff.

My greatest fear is saying something to one of my female students that could be construed as sexual harassment. Nearly all of my students are female. One little comment about how they look and my career could be over. Further, several of my students know this. A couple have even demanded higher grades than what they earned. One told me that if I didn't give her an A, she would tell people that I hit on her and touched her breasts.

I am well aware of this peril and I know there is nothing that I can do about it. It is very hard, if not impossible, to disprove lies. All I can do is relax and not worry about such things until they occur. Then if they occur, I will count on my two or three close friends for emotional support.

My main advocate is my girlfriend, who wants to be called "Daisey." How she can put up with me, I don't know. I couldn't be half as happy or as "successful" without her.

Far more than anybody else in my life, she has made a huge effort to understand everything about me and ADHD. She reads my books and constantly asks questions about what life is like from my perspective. She might not understand why I do stupid things, but she genuinely thinks that my oddities are endearing—at least, she does most of the time.

There have been many times when my ADHD gets in the way of our relationship. For example, when I am really hyperactive, I can't be hugged. When she put her arms around me, I feel very confined and claustrophobic. I have to get away. She says that she understands, but I think that she sometimes takes it personally.

I also have problems listening to her once in a while. This is especially problematic when we are about to get into an argument. I try to focus on what she is telling me, but I can't. Further, I can't pretend to be paying attention. My eyes wander and I start looking bored, which gets her even angrier.

As with past relationships, I do a lot of stupid things around Daisey. Last week, we got into a huge fight because I walked out of a store without holding the door open in front of her. The door slammed in her face.

I also say things that I don't mean. For instance, yesterday I was telling her how terrific she is. I wanted to say that she is so thoughtful and selfless. But what ended up coming out of my mouth was that she was "thoughtless." A few days before, I tried explaining how much I loved being around her and how I always enjoy her company. But what I actually said was, "I rarely dread being with you." Such comments have been coined "Robisms." She usually just laughs at them and repeats them at parties.

Fortunately, these incidents are becoming fewer and further between. She is very supportive and has developed a kind of "ADHD radar." Right when I am starting to get hyperactive or distracted or inattentive, she redirects me. If we are cuddling on the couch and I begin vibrating, she will make me get up and take the dogs for a walk. Or we will go work out. Moreover, she has a really good grasp of what I can and can't do. She doesn't expect me to sit down through entire movies or make constant eye contact during conversations. Like I said, she is incredible!

All in all, the present is a pretty great place. I can't think of anything to improve it, not even a million dollars or a Pulitzer (although both would be nice). My present is clearly far better than my past. But I realize my past is how I got to the present, so I try not to think too negatively of it. Yes, ADHD has been a pain in the ass sometimes—but, overall, it has helped me get to where I am and, as I have said, I like the view from where I am now standing. As Jimmy Stewart found out, it really is a wonderful life.

The question that you probably are having is, "How did you get to where you are?" This is a good question. It is also the primary reason for this entire exploration.

Shortly after being diagnosed with ADHD, I was watching an infomercial about some miracle product that was guaranteed to make people more energetic. The spokesperson stated that energetic people have better lives than the sluggards of the world. For proof, viewers were shown on one side of the television screen a hard-working, attractive man getting promoted, being the life of the party, and smiling. On the other side of the television screen, a less-than-attractive man with his hair and tie in disarray was sitting behind a messy desk trying to stay awake. He wasn't getting promoted, going to parties, or acting very happy. If he had only bought these magical, all-natural pills, the slob would have everything that he wanted in life.

As I watched this program, I had a kind of epiphany. It occurred to me that there was this big "self-help" industry trying to make people more energetic, creative, and to "think outside of the box." I realized that these were the natural characteristics of ADHD! By definition, people with ADHD are very active and creative. We may have problems paying attention, but it struck me that there were ways of correcting this problem. In fact, there had to be ways of taking all of this energy that people with ADHD have and turning it into periods of extreme productivity. Since seeing the infomercial, I have made an effort to find ways of making ADHD a gift. It has been my professional and personal quest ever since.

In addition to reading everything on ADHD that I could get my hands on, I began thinking about what was effective for me. I joined support groups, such as CHADD, and listened to what worked for other people. I then experimented with different strategies in a very systematic way.

I kept a little notepad and pencil in my back pocket. Whenever an idea about how I could become more productive or attentive came to me, I wrote it down before I could forget. I kept journals of what was helpful and what wasn't. Moreover, I constantly tried to ascertain why various strategies worked for me and why some didn't. I took data on my performance and monitored my overall day-to-day moods. Through my efforts, I developed many effective strategies for making ADHD an asset.

These strategies fall predominantly into three key categories. The first involves making my environments more conducive to having ADHD. These strategies will be discussed in the next chapter. The other two areas involve learning how to learn more efficiently and methods of supporting myself emotionally. These strategies will be summarized in chapters 13 and 14, respectively. I hope that they help you.

⑫

STRATEGIES FOR CHANGING MY ENVIRONMENTS

Environmental factors involve those things immediately around me that influence how I behave. At first, I focused on factors that made it challenging for me to concentrate, then I attempted to identify variables that helped me calm down and focus.

Through a great deal of self-reflection and observation, I realized that my behavior was largely influenced by my surroundings. For example, I can't concentrate when there is too much or too little noise. Further, there are certain sounds or sound patterns that are especially distracting. Specifically, high-pitched noises, such as the voices of little children, cut right through me. It doesn't matter how loud or soft they are. If something is high-pitched, it automatically grabs my attention and yanks it away from what I am attempting to focus on.

Whispers especially drive me crazy. Even if I can't hear what people are saying, the sound of them whispering is extremely distracting. It is like nails on a chalkboard. I can almost feel my ears "turn" toward the noise, like radar, and no matter how hard I try I can't turn them back to the task at hand.

Periodic sound also gets me off task. I can normally deal with the steady drone of clatter, but not a noise followed by a silence followed by a few more noises and then silence and so on. As a result, I have never been able to work well at libraries. It isn't that it is too quiet, it is that there are subtle, infrequent sounds. Somebody will cough. Somebody will shift in a chair. Somebody will exhale or sigh. I can hear the air conditioner kick on and off. I hear everything and every time that I hear something new, part of my attention gets pulled away. With this in mind, I began looking for places where I could study effectively. They had to be not so quiet that I could hear everything, but also where the din was fairly continuous.

Like I said, libraries are usually no good for me. I can study outside, but only if the noises around me are fairly constant. In other words, I could study by a highway, where there is a continuous buzz of cars. But I couldn't study by a residential street where a car would go by every five or ten minutes.

Trying to find an environment with the right sounds was difficult, so I began experimenting with creating various background noises that could help me focus. For example, I would go to the library with a Walkman and tapes of my favorite music. This didn't work very well. I hated having the earphones on. The pressure on my ears gave me headaches. Further, whenever I moved, I could hear the "crinkling" of the foam ear pads. It really bothered me.

Moreover, while I love the Beatles, I can't listen to them and study at the same time. I got too caught up in the lyrics or the beat of the bass or the memories that the songs bring to mind. So rather than listening to my favorite music, I started listening to things that I neither liked nor hated. For instance, as I write this, I am listening to a CD called *Bach at Bedtime*. While I am not a big fan of the classics, the soft flowing movement of the orchestra not only calms my mind but it also drowns out the noise from the cars driving by and the people walking down the hallway.

I have a stack of various calming CDs. Some have music, such as the classics or Chicago Blues. Others have nature sounds, such as rainstorms or birds chirping. Further, I seem to go in cycles as to what is most effective. Currently, I am on a classics kick. I pop in Bach and I can concentrate. Two weeks ago, I could only listen to soft jazz, John Coltrane in particular. While one CD might work wonderfully one day, it may drive me crazy the next. So I try to keep a wide range of options wherever I work.

The common thread between all of these CDs is that the sound is soft, slow, and relaxing. It also helps if it doesn't vary much in pitch or intensity. I need something that will flow through me and sink into my head, but not to such a degree that I can't think of anything else. After a while, I will have the CD on and I will not "hear" it anymore. It is still playing, but I will not notice it. I certainly notice when it goes off, however, so I usually put the CDs on constant play mode. I play the same CD over and over again, sometimes for days on end.

In addition to playing CDs, I also have a fish tank in my office. The low hum of the air pump and the soft gurgling of the bubbles calm me. For a while, I didn't even have fish in the tank. I just liked the sound it made.

When I work at home, I typically have the television on. Some of the same principles seem to apply. I can't have anything on that is too interesting or else I will watch it more than I want to. Further, it can't be too loud or variable. Baseball games are pretty good for me to work by. If I get distracted, I can glance up, see the score, and then return to grading papers or writing. Old sitcoms, such as *Hogan's Heroes* or *MASH*, are also effective, but they have to be episodes that I have seen over and over again. They have to be slightly boring, but not annoying. I have to be able to look up and think, "Oh yeah, I remember that part" and then go back to work knowing the entire next scene by heart.

I should point out that I tried earplugs. They are really good for blocking out all noises, but I had the same problem as I did with the Walkman. The plugs felt strange in my ears and distracted me. Maybe if I wore them more often, the sensation of having something in my ears would be less bothersome.

In addition to sound, I soon realized that visual stimuli can also be very distracting. This is especially true if there is movement. I think that this is why I always sit in the back whenever I attend classes or conferences or go to the movies. When there are people behind me, I can sense them stirring. It is very unsettling. Further, I feel compelled to turn around, which gets me off task even more. Plus, it looks rude if I keep turning and staring at them. For these reasons, I usually advise teachers to put kids with ADHD in the back corners of the classroom where all the stimuli are in front of them. Otherwise, they will be turning around to see what is going on.

I have tried working while sitting in carrels but I am not able to concentrate there. The same is true when I use the small study rooms at the library. The dirty-white bare walls of the study rooms drove me crazy. Sounds echoed and I felt the opposite of claustrophobic, if that makes sense. In fact, I cannot teach in some of the classrooms at my university. The walls are unadorned and are the same colors as the floor and the ceiling. I simply can't concentrate when I am in them.

Just as I can't concentrate when there is too much going on around me, I cannot focus effectively when there is too little stimulation. Being in a completely bare room with bright walls would make me insane even more than being in Grand Central Station during rush hour. I had to find a comfortable middle ground.

After extensive experimenting, I found that I concentrated best when I had a lot of things around me but the visual stimuli couldn't be too novel. For instance, the room where I was initially tested for ADHD had loads of interesting objects around me. There were dozens of cartoons taped to the walls, toys all over the floor, and bookshelves full of neat knickknacks. I felt compelled to look at all of them before I could work. If everything in the room had been familiar to me, I wouldn't have been distracted. But if there were no stimuli at all, my brain seemed to look for it, which is why I can't concentrate in empty or spartan rooms.

During my search for strategies to make myself more productive, I also realized that I don't like clean environments. As a child, I always said that I didn't like my desk clean. At the time I was probably just making an excuse not to be neat and orderly. But as I experimented, I found that I couldn't concentrate when everything around me is "organized." I need clutter. I need piles of rubbish around me. I need filth.

As I look around my office while I write this, I can see crap heaped up all around me. I am not kidding when I say that the fire marshal has been into my office twice and demanded that I clear a pathway to the door. Like I said earlier, my colleagues and students, and even some people I do not know, find it necessary to pop their heads in my office and make rude comments about what a slob I am. I am a slob. I admit it, but I have tried to be neat and it doesn't work for me for several reasons.

First, being neat takes a tremendous amount of time and attention to detail. I don't like wasting my time cleaning because I know that in a couple of days everything will be messy again. I find the whole process very frustrating and avoid it as much as I can. Further, after I clean, I can never remember where I put everything. So, not only do I waste time cleaning, but I also waste more time trying to find what I have supposedly organized.

More important, when I am working in my office, I am surrounded by relaxing stimuli. The piles of paper, stacks of books, and general debris all around me aren't distracting. Actually, the clutter is very comforting, kind of like being wrapped in a warm blanket on a cold day. When I clean, everything is in a different space, so it is like being in a new environment. The old clutter rearranged now distracts me because I am not used to seeing things in their new places.

Of course, some people will see this as an excuse for being a slob. Perhaps it is. However, my answer to them is this. Would you prefer me to be cleaner, but less productive, or have a dirty office and be more prolific? By and large, with the exception of the fire marshal, people usually see my point.

When I give workshops on ADHD, I almost always have a parent or teacher complaining about a child with ADHD who is messy. They say, "His desk is hemorrhaging paper!" or "Her bed is covered with dirty clothes!" They then beg me to give them some sort of magical solution to make their child neater.

The first thing that I ask these beleaguered adults is, "Why is it so important that you can see your child's bed?" "Why is so important that papers are neatly organized in their desk?" The parents and teachers usually respond by saying that kids should be neat, or that he is not cleaning because he is trying to be disobedient, or that her schoolwork suffers because she can't find anything.

The only reason to help a child be neater is the last one—to help him do his schoolwork. Who cares if you have dirty underwear on your bed or your desk is messy? Isn't being happy, healthy, and able to learn more important than what others think of you?

Whenever I say such things, I see parents and teachers cringe. They have been brought up with the notion that things must be in their places before work can begin. Further, the Judeo-Christian "cleanliness is next to godliness" principle is well engrained into our psyche.

Please don't get me wrong. Being neat and tidy certainly is important. But I believe that parents and teachers should think about why they are trying to force a child to go against his or her natural tendencies. Is it because "everybody should be neat"? Or is it because "students lose their work and cannot concentrate in their cluttered environments"? If a child can be productive with a messy desk or bedroom, I say leave him alone. The only exception that I can think of is if the clutter is causing a health hazard. Obviously, if rats are breeding underneath a child's bed, a thorough cleaning probably is in order. Still, far too much emphasis and time is placed on making people with ADHD like non-ADHD people. Instead, I think that the emphasis should be on productivity and emotional well-being.

As I have said before, I need an environment that has constant noise and plenty of familiar visual stimuli. But I also need a certain kind of lighting to be able to think clearly. It can't be too bright or too dim. The wrong kind of lighting prevents me from sitting still and concentrating.

When playing with different types of lighting for my work environments, I stumbled across some interesting findings. For instance, I tend to prefer dark rooms to bright ones—the darker, the better. As long as I have enough light by which to see, I am fine. But the key is the type of light by which I am working.

Fluorescent lights are horrible for me. They hurt my eyes and give me headaches. Further, they buzz and vibrate in an unpleasant way. Next time you stand under a bank of fluorescent lights, stop and listen. You can hear them buzzing. It is very faint, but immensely annoying. Further, I can feel them vibrating. It is like I can feel the waves of light bouncing off me. It is extremely challenging to concentrate when fluorescent lights are the only lights in the room.

You would think that sunlight would be the best for me, but it isn't. The light itself is fine. But whenever it is bright and sunny out, I want to stop working and go outside. It is very taxing to get anything done during nice days. As a result, *when* I work (e.g., in the evenings or night) is as important as *where* I work, as we will discuss later.

The best lighting for me comes from full-spectrum light bulbs. They are expensive, so I don't use them everywhere, just in my offices at work and home. From what I understand, they simulate the rays of the sun without the burning radiation. People who have reptiles as pets use these lights because they give animals various vitamins. They have also been used to treat depression, which could explain why I like them.

Of course, normal incandescent lights work almost as well, but they have to be fairly dim. The one that I am using now is forty watts. Further, they have to be "soft white." Other light bulbs are too bright and harsh.

My favorite light sources are candles. Learning this has helped me a great deal. There is something about a candle that allows me to focus my attention almost immediately. The soft, slowly flickering flame soothes me. When I have a couple of lit candles around, I feel relaxed yet motivated to work.

Further, I buy scented candles. The one that is burning now is vanilla. The smell is very sweet and refreshing, but not overwhelming. Much like the flickering light it produces, the smell calms me down. They work so well that I buy them in bulk.

There are two problems with using candles. The first is that I can't read by them—they aren't bright enough. Second, I frequently leave them burning unattended. Many times I have gone home only to realize later that I left the candle burning back in my office. Given the massive amount of papers and flammable materials piled in and around my desk, a rogue candle could burn down the entire building! So this is a serious issue.

After a great deal of systematic investigation, I have been able to create an environment that is pretty conducive for working. I am not saying that I can be productive all the time, but I can certainly stay seated and focused in these environments far longer and better than any other places. Let me take a minute and describe my office to you.

The room is probably eight feet wide and twelve feet long. The floor is tiled, but is mostly covered with papers, stacks of books, and general debris, including dirty Kleenexes, empty Tupperware containers that used to have my lunch in them, and popcorn crumbs. Like I said, I know that I am a slob but I am happy the way I am, so leave me alone.

The walls are creamy white in color, which normally would bother my eyes, but I have covered them with pieces of paper. Anything that is important gets taped to the wall in front of me. For instance, to my right is my class schedule. To my left is a piece of paper that reminds me that I am in control of my thoughts and beliefs (it is kind of an inspirational sign for me). Behind me are pictures of my friends, family, and dogs from the Humane Society that I have trained. There is also a big framed picture of Stuart Sutcliffe, who was one of the original Beatles. He serves as a source of inspiration for me as well.

To my right is a desk, but I never use it. It is covered with papers and books a couple feet high. Actually, other than the drawers and the legs, you can't see the desk at all. The drawers are open and reveal their odd contents, such as a half-eaten bag of popcorn, a five-pound bag of sugar (which I use to sweeten tea), dirty plastic forks and spoons, and copies of various articles and papers. There might even be a few assignments from students that I thought that I had lost.

To my left is an eight-foot-high metal bookshelf that has four books lying on their sides. The rest of the shelves are covered with papers, plastic bags, CDs, plastic cups, empty cardboard boxes, dirty dishes, a stuffed animal given to me as a gift, and tea bags (not yet used; the used tea bags are piled on the floor by the door. I generally miss when I throw them at the trashcan.)

Directly in front of me is my computer, which sits on a two-tiered computer table. In addition to the computer, the table is covered with papers, pictures of my students, several empty yogurt containers, a cup of now-cold tea (mango-Ceylon flavored), various pens and pencils, a bottle of aspirin, a bottle of vitamins, an empty bottle that once had contact lens solution, a burned-out light bulb, a phone, a three-wick vanilla scented candle, a laptop computer upon which I am currently playing a game, and a mountain of other crap.

On the floor immediately around me is a box of corn flakes, piles of papers that I need to grade, a bag of oranges, books (including *The Lord of the Rings* by J. R. R. Tolkien), several pennies, popcorn, paperclips, fish food, and a roll of tape. If I move my feet more than six inches in any direction, I will step on something.

It is 12:06 in the afternoon. The shades are drawn over my window, although a little of the Wisconsin winter sun is able to peek into the room. The overhead fluorescent lights are off and the only other illumination in the room comes from the computer screen, the vanilla-scented candle, and a floor lamp.

The floor lamp is very important. It has a long, bendable neck that enables me to project light on top of my keyboard like an arrow that constantly points me to what I should be doing. It is a great natural cue that redirects my attention back to my keyboard. Everything other than my keyboard is relatively dark.

I have a fish tank on my desk. I can hear the hum of the filter and the bubbling of the water. I am also listening to a CD of Native American flutes. Bach started to bother me so I put on a different CD.

And I am sitting on a pillow on a chair with good lower back support and arm rests. A comfortable chair is really important to me. In fact, when I accepted my current position, I negotiated to have a new chair. I can't concentrate if I am uncomfortable. How teachers expect their students, with and without ADHD, to work while sitting on those hard school chairs is beyond me.

I have covered the window on my office door with paper, so nobody can see in. This keeps me from getting distracted when people walk by. It also keeps visitors to a minimum. Since they can't see in, and I normally don't have my overhead lights on, they just naturally assume that I am not in my office so they leave me alone!

So there you have it—my office. It might sound like a filthy pigsty, and it is, but it is the best place for me to work and think. Over the past ten months, I have written three books and two articles in this office. I couldn't have been as productive any other place.

I should also take some time to talk about my home environment, especially in regard to my bedroom. You see, when I was younger I would fall asleep as soon as my energy ran out. I would collapse on my bed and be asleep within moments.

As I entered my adolescence, and even more so as an adult, falling asleep became problematic. Up until a couple years ago, it would usually take me a couple of hours to fall asleep every night. I could be exhausted physically, but my mind wouldn't turn off. I would lie awake in bed, tossing and turning, with my many thoughts spinning out of control and keeping me awake. I thought that this was just how it was for everybody. I thought that it took everybody several hours to fall asleep. But then I learned that most people fall asleep after only seven to twelve minutes.

My difficulties sleeping aren't uncommon. As many as half of adults with ADHD also have sleeping disorders, such as chronic insomnia. Sometimes this is the result of the medications that they take. Other times, it is because they simply can't turn off their mind.

When I began planning my first book on ADHD, I decided to include a section on the sleeping problems that people with ADHD typically experience. I researched the topic and found many strategies that doctors say are suppose to help people sleep better. I tried some of them and they helped me immensely. I now fall asleep relatively quickly. I doubt if I remain awake more than fifteen or twenty minutes after lying down. Further, I sleep more soundly and feel more refreshed in the mornings than I ever did before.

The most important suggestion that I found in the literature involved preparing to go to sleep. Unfortunately, I, like most people with ADHD, don't spend much time relaxing. I am constantly doing something. If I am not writing or grading papers, I am either working out or walking the dogs at the Humane Society. Moreover, I am always thinking and planning things out in my head. When I decide to go to bed, my mind is not ready to turn itself off and I would lie awake for a long while.

According to what I have read, people should not simply stop what they are doing and go to bed. They need to prepare their mind and body for sleep. For instance, people should sit and relax for at least a half an hour before lying down. Further, they should not read or watch anything that gets them excited, otherwise they will not be relaxed. This is why I don't watch the news before I go to bed. It is too upsetting for me. If I do, I lie awake in my bed thinking about all of the horrible things going on in the world.

In addition to not watching or reading anything that would heighten your emotional state, you should also not exercise or do any strenuous activities right before bed. The last thing people should do as they are preparing to sleep is to increase their pulse. They should relax and unwind.

This was good for me to learn. I used to do sit-ups and work out right before I got ready for bed, which probably contributed to my insomnia. Lately, I have been working out in the morning. This wakes me up and starts my day on a positive note. It also minimizes my hyperactivity.

I also learned that people should go to sleep roughly at the same time each day. Before I found this out, I would try to go to sleep at various hours, depending upon what day it was. For instance, when I had to teach a morning class, I would go to bed about 10:00 P.M. the night before. But if I were teaching mainly night classes, I would stay up well past midnight writing. Further, on weekends, I would go to bed whenever the mood struck me.

Now, I go to bed and wake up roughly at the same time every day. This has helped enormously. Not only do I fall asleep more quickly, but I also wake up without my alarm clock.

A couple years ago, I started using meditation to prepare me for sleep. Because I can't sit still for long, I am not very good at it. Still, the act of closing my eyes and allowing my many thoughts to drift in and out of my consciousness enables me to relax.

As with my office, changing my sleeping environment has been very useful. For instance, the light from my clock is distracting. Plus, watching the minutes slowly slip by produces a lot of anxiety for me. The more time passes, the greater my anxieties grow. The more anxious I become, the harder it is for me to calm my mind and drift off. So I turned my alarm clock to face the wall. Now it doesn't bother me.

Additionally, I listen to background noise when I am falling asleep. I have a CD player that has a continuous play program so the CD continues throughout the night. Selecting the proper "mood" music took some time. It has to be soft without any sudden changes in pitch or volume, such as ocean waves or a gentle thunderstorm. The sound of the rolling surf or the pitter-patter of the rain is perfect for helping me settle down. It also drowns out the nightly noises that keep me up, such as cars driving by my window or my cats playing on the stairs outside my bedroom door.

As with trying to read when I can't concentrate, I have learned not to force going to sleep. If I can't fall asleep within a half hour or so, I get up and watch some mindless television show. I found that lying in bed, trying to will myself to relax, just makes matters worse.

Moreover, rather than attempting to compel my mind into calming down, I simply let it run away. As I relax, listening to the ocean's waves, I let my mind go where it will without any guidance from me. If I try to actively clear my mind, I find myself wrestling with my thoughts, which clutters my mind even further and prevents me from sinking into a deep sleep.

Perhaps the most surprising tip that I found in the literature involves the use of the bed and bedroom. Apparently, if people use their bedroom for anything other than sleeping, they increase the chances of having insomnia. This makes sense. If you only sleep on your bed, your body will think when you lie down, "Ah, it must be time to sleep!" But if you sometimes lie on your bed reading or watching television, your body will get confused. In other words, your body becomes conditioned to fall asleep when sleeping is the only thing that it does when it is in the bedroom. When I stopped reading and watching television in bed, I began falling asleep much quicker.

So there you have it. A lot of my success is the result of manipulating various variables and creating environments that are conducive to being productive. I should point out that these strategies work best when used together. Further, after I started using them for a while, my brain seemed to become conditioned. Now, when I sit with a fresh cup of steaming hot tea in my office with all of the lights off, except my floor lamp shining down on the keyboard and a flickering candle, and I hear soft music playing in the background, my mind calms down and I am able to focus.

I am not saying that there aren't times when I can't concentrate. There are. Sometimes, I can't focus enough to read or write. It is just that these times are becoming less frequent or prolonged. Additionally, when I am able to concentrate, I have developed some very effective strategies for enhancing my learning, which will be discussed in the next chapter.

⓭

STRATEGIES FOR
LEARNING TO LEARN

Figuring out how to change my environment so that I can sit still and concentrate was the first step in improving my life. I also had to learn how to learn. I am still in the process of identifying strategies that are effective for me, but here is what I have come up with thus far.

The most important thing is knowing when to work and when not to. This actually involves a number of different skills and dispositions. Let me explain.

If you hand most people a newspaper and ask them to read it, they usually can right there on the spot. Moreover, they probably could explain what they have read (provided that the article is within their reading level). People with ADHD can't always do this. Sometimes we are so distractible that we simply cannot read or write or think clearly. It isn't that we aren't trying, it's just that sometimes our minds don't function the way that we want them to.

For instance, many times students will come up to me and ask if I can proofread one of their assignments. Often, I tell them that I can't. It isn't because I don't have the time or that I don't want to help, it is just that sometimes I can't focus enough to be able to read. I can say the words out loud, but I can't string them together into a coherent sentence.

I can usually limit the frequency and the intensity of my "brain dead" days by exercising regularly and getting a good night's sleep. If I can't focus enough to read or think effectively, I jump on a Stairmaster for ten minutes and I am cured! Sometimes, I will run up and down the stairs at school. All it takes is elevating my heart rate just a little bit for a few minutes and my mind becomes clear as a bell.

The worst thing that I can do when I can't concentrate is attempt to force it. The harder I try, the more I struggle. The more I struggle, the more frustrated I get and the harder it is for me to focus. It is a very tight spiral. Understanding this was an important lesson. If I can't do something, I don't try to do it then. I wait, do something else, and then try again later.

Finding times when I am able to be productive was another important step in being able to learn effectively. This took some trial and error, but I found that I could generally concentrate better either in the early morning or in the evening. I have a hard time working during the day, especially when it is really nice out. I can do it, but it is much easier to focus in the mornings and evenings when everything is very calm and quiet. I can sit at my desk and not be distracted by all of the noise outside of my window or people going here and there.

Recently, I have been getting up around 5:30 in the morning. I walk my dog, which is a wonderful way to exercise and clear my mind, and then work from about 6:30 A.M. to 10:30 A.M. Around 10:30, I start losing my ability to maintain my attention, so I go work out at the YMCA, eat lunch, and when I come back, I am good for another few hours.

I used to work from 7:00 in the evening to well past midnight. Once I remember working on a manuscript all through the night. When I looked up from my computer, I thought that the sun was setting. I thought to myself, "Boy! I am getting a lot done in such a short period of time!" But really the sun was rising. I had worked through the entire night without even realizing it!

Of course, as I have gotten older, staying up to all hours is less appealing. I need to have a consistent bedtime and get my six hours of sleep or I am dead the next day. So I have pretty much stuck to working in the early mornings.

Because I can't "perform on command," I had to learn that I shouldn't procrastinate. As much as it is my natural character, I cannot allow myself to put off until tomorrow what I can do today. If I do things as soon as I can, right when I am thinking about them, I lessen the chances of forgetting what I need to do. Further, I also decrease the chance that I will come up against a deadline only to find that I can't concentrate enough to do the task.

Learning not to procrastinate wasn't easy. I still do it from time to time, but I am much better now than before. The trick is to keep a record of everything that needs to be done and by when. I have a day planner in which I write down *everything* that needs to be remembered (e.g., meetings, tasks, social outings). Further, the people around me know that if I don't write things down, I will forget them, so they will frequently remind me.

I had two difficulties when I first started using a day planner. The first was not losing it. To prevent me from misplacing it, I got the biggest planner that I could find. Those small, pocket-sized ones get hidden too easily under the piles of crap in my office. I also get planners with brightly colored covers. This helps them stand out in my office. Further, I keep the planner where I need it, which is usually next to my computer. Whenever I can't find it, I check there first. Ninety percent of the time, it is within arm's reach of my chair in my office.

Another problem that I had using daily planners is remembering to check them regularly. Fortunately, this is where ADHD actually helps me. As I said before, people with ADHD are inclined to have addictive personalities. We abuse drugs and alcohol more often than do non-ADHDers. We also fall in and out of love very quickly. It seems that this propensity for addiction stems from our need for constant action and stimulation. Again, we tend to be very active. So what better way to use that hyperactivity than to create positive routines? In other words, I have gotten into the habit of checking my daily planner as soon as I sit down at my computer in the morning and just before I leave my office for the day. It is almost like a compulsion. If I have to be doing a dozen different things all at once, I can make one of those things checking my day planner.

I can't say enough about developing positive routines. "Addiction" has a bad rap, but I have learned to use it to my advantage. For instance, in addition to checking my daily planner, I am addicted to working out. Every morning, I get up and jump on my elliptical exercise machine for fifteen minutes. I can't seem to have a good day without exercising at least a little bit right after getting up. It clears my mind and calms my body.

I am also addicted to journaling. Throughout the day, usually before I go to bed, I have to write down some of my thoughts. This enables me to let go of the ideas that buzz around my head. Without doing this, my mind keeps spinning out of control and it takes me a couple hours to fall asleep.

I suppose that I am also addicted to writing books. As soon as I finish one manuscript, I have to start another. I genuinely do not feel good if I am not writing about something. As result, I have been fairly successful professionally.

By utilizing my energy in positive recurring ways, I have turned the "evil hyperactivity" into a valuable tool. But how did I get into the habit of doing something so regularly that it became a good habit? It took some work and a lot of support from my friends, but I did it!

For instance, in the past, I habitually lost my car keys. Nearly every morning, I would be late for work because it took me a half an hour to find my keys. In fact, sometimes I had to ride my bike to work because I couldn't find them. So what did I do?

The first thing that I did was to identify a good place to put my keys. When I get out of my car and enter the house, I go through the kitchen. The first thing that I come to in the kitchen is the dishwasher. On top of the dishwasher is the best place for my keys because it is in the open and I can find the keys easily.

To get into the habit of leaving my keys in the same spot every day, I placed a Post-it note on the dishwasher that said in big letters "PUT KEYS HERE!" The problem is, after a while, I would start ignoring the reminder. So, I would keep putting new signs on different colored Post-its. The act of rewriting the notes, as well as seeing a new message every couple of days, kept me actively thinking about where I was supposed to set my keys.

Now it is a force of habit. I don't even think about it anymore. I walk in and drop my keys on the dishwasher. I no longer need the prompts to do it.

I did something very similar with checking my daily planner in the morning. I programmed my computer to flash a message that read "CHECK YOUR DAILY PLANNER" as soon as I turned it on. So every morning, I had a visual reminder what I was supposed to do. Further, my computer would not allow me to continue doing anything else until I clicked on the daily planner prompt.

Things that don't occur very frequently are a bit harder to develop into routines. For example, I often forget birthdays. After all, they only come around once a year. Fortunately, my girlfriend seems to find great joy in reminding me about sending birthday cards out. At the beginning of every month she asks me, "Are there any birthdays this month?" I stop and think and say, "Yea, so-and-so has a birthday." To which she replies, "Then write it down right now. Put it in your date book." Moreover, whenever I get a new day planner, I try to go through the old one and copy down all the anniversaries and birthdays from the previous year.

I also use computer programs to remind me about sporadic events, such as meetings and outings. I have arranged it so that I get e-mails from myself a week, five days, and two days before important events. Since I am always in my office working and have my e-mail up and running, I never miss the messages.

Remembering meetings is also very problematic for me. I have meetings nearly every day, but at different times and in different rooms. As soon as I get an e-mail about a meeting, I print it out, and make a notation in my daily planner. I then tape the printed e-mail to my wall right next to my computer.

Even with all of my computer programs and visual prompts, I know that I will forget things. I have a horrible memory. So I have to write things down as soon as I think of them.

When preparing to write this book, I brainstormed a list of the stories and events that I wanted to talk about. But I knew that I didn't come up with everything, so I keep a little notebook with a golf pencil in my back pocket. Whenever I thought of another story to tell or strategy to discuss, I wrote it down right away.

Another strategy is breaking tasks down into very small units. Even when I write, I don't say to myself, "I want to write an entire chapter today." Instead, I set much more manageable goals. If I write a couple of good paragraphs in one sitting, I am happy. If I expect more than that, I will only disappoint myself and get frustrated. Again, preventing frustration is the key for me to be productive! If I get stressed, I can't function.

I also do a bunch of different things all at once. For example, as I am sitting in my office writing this, I am also grading quizzes from one of my classes as well as playing a computer game on my laptop computer, which is to my immediate left. I write a few sentences, and when I begin losing my train of thought, I grade one quiz, and then play the game for thirty seconds or so. I keep going back and forth. It may sound hectic, but it keeps my mind from getting bored.

Additionally, I am currently writing two other books. When I get stuck on this one, I move on to a different project. If I try forcing my attention on any one task, I usually get bogged down and depressed. When I can't concentrate on something, it is no use struggling with it. So I move on to something else and then come back to the first task after my head has settled down a bit.

Hyperactivity has always been an issue for me. From being my mother's "little monster" to getting spanked for not sitting on the story rug to having problems professionally because I fidget during meetings, being overly active has caused its share of difficulties. For instance, on more than one occasion I have been watching a movie at a theater. Somebody from ten seats down will come up and ask me to stop bouncing my knee, which I do a great deal. Apparently my knee bouncing shook the entire row. So I politely apologize and sit still. Within minutes, if not seconds, my knee started bouncing again on its own. People get really upset and have even thrown popcorn at me.

This kind of excessive movement is classic ADHD. If it is not knees bouncing, it is hair twirling, finger tapping, or something equally annoying. We have to keep moving. It is one of the most common complaints that teachers have about their students with ADHD.

Regrettably, teachers and parents frequently try coercing children with ADHD to stop moving. Then when the child fails to do so, adults see it as a "willful disregard for the rules" or "disrespecting authority figures." But this usually isn't the case.

Expelling energy is a biological necessity. Everybody has it. Just imagine being cooped up in a car all day during a long trip. After a while, it is probably hard for even "normal" people to remain motionless. People with ADHD have the same problem, but it is magnified many times over. We simply can't always sit without moving for long.

The best way that I can explain hyperactivity is to imagine that you have a bad itchy rash. Maybe you have poison ivy or a bug bite. Imagine trying not to scratch despite the overwhelming urge to do so. As long as you concentrate, you probably can stop yourself from scratching. But as soon as you think about something else, you would start scratching without even thinking about it.

Hyperactivity for people with ADHD is much like scratching. Yes, we can control it, but only to a point. If I harness all of my attention and will, I can stop my leg from bouncing. But as soon as I go back to doing whatever, such as watching a movie or paying attention to the teacher, it starts bouncing again on its own. I cannot count the number of times I have upset people because I would say that I would sit still, but then couldn't.

Remember, everybody has a biological need to expel energy. People with ADHD just have more energy to expel. So the question really shouldn't be "How do I make this kid sit still?" I have fought that battle my entire life and I usually lose. Instead, the question should be two-fold: "How can I get this kid to utilize his energy in a more appropriate manner?" and "How can I minimize the disruptions caused by this kid's energy?"

I have thought about these two questions a great deal. Like I said, I have attempted to force myself to sit still, but no matter how hard I try, I cannot completely repress my hyperactivity for long. Although I am still working on harnessing my energy, I have developed several strategies that have benefited me tremendously.

First, as I mentioned earlier, regular exercise has decreased my hyperactivity dramatically. Even running up and down a few flights of steps enables me to sit still at least for a little while.

Another strategy that I have developed is wiggling my toes. Wiggling my toes allows me to expel energy in a way that doesn't bother anybody else. Try it. Can you see that your toes are moving? Probably not if you have shoes on. Further, even if somebody could see your toes moving, they most likely would not be as distracted as if you were bouncing your knee or tapping your finger.

Sometimes I simply cannot sit down. It is physically painful to be on my butt. I can't explain it other than referring back to the itching analogy. Scratching an itch feels good; not scratching an itch produces a certain degree of pain. Perhaps "pain" is not quite the right word. Maybe "discomfort" is closer to the mark. Whatever you call it, it isn't a pleasant feeling.

The same is true for people with ADHD who try sitting still when their bodies don't want to. It is very uncomfortable remaining seated when I am in a hyperactive phase. This is rather challenging when I have long departmental meetings. Sometimes they can go on for two or three hours and I simply am not able to stay in my seat for that long.

One of the things that I do is to kneel rather than sit. It sounds kind of strange, but instead of sitting at the conference table, I kneel beside it. It gets me off of my butt, which feels good. Plus, when I am kneeling, I am roughly the same height as when I am sitting, so most people don't even realize that I am out of my seat.

Of course, taking breaks is also very helpful. I frequently excuse myself from meetings, walk to the water fountain, and then come back and sit down. That usually buys me a little more time and allows me to focus my attention better when I come back.

Sometimes I can't leave meetings, especially when something important is being discussed. In such circumstances, I get up and stand behind everybody. At first I felt like I was distracting my colleagues, but they seem to understand now. Some of them actually get up and stand, too. People with ADHD are not the only people who have trouble sitting down for long periods of time!

One of the primary problems that students with ADHD have academically is that we often do not know what or how to study. For example, just as visual stimuli divert our attention, we also get distracted by all of the information that teachers present. We often don't know what information is important and what is filler material.

The best class that I took during my college days was on study skills. It was wonderful! It taught me how to take organized notes that made sense weeks later. I also learned how to identify key topics and supporting details and how to summarize ideas rather than recording what the teacher said word for word. I highly recommend such courses.

Learning to read textbooks was also a critical skill. Too many of my students read their textbooks as if they were reading a novel. That is, they start at the beginning of the chapter and read each word until they get to the end. This is a huge waste of time.

When reading a textbook, students should first skim the chapter. They should look at the title, pictures, and the headings. Then they should guess what is being discussed and recognize common themes or words. Rather than just reading the words, they should actively ask themselves "What is the author trying to tell me?" and "What is important here?" Once they have a good idea what the chapter is about, they should read the introduction and summary. If there is anything that they don't understand, they should read the portion of the chapter that covers that topic. Further, they should answer any study questions found at the beginning or end of the chapter. A fifty-page chapter could easily be read in about ten to fifteen minutes.

I use very similar strategies to help me pay attention to people. For instance, I listen actively. I picture what they are talking about and anticipate what is going to be said next. I also repeat key phrases and summarize main points in my head.

My difficulty with paying attention often hinders my ability to remember people's names. I have an awful memory and some people get offended when I forget who they are, especially when I have been interacting with them for a while or if I am on an interview or date.

Lately, I have been trying a strategy that somebody suggested. It appears to be working. Basically, when people tell me their name, I repeat it three times to myself and once out loud. For instance, I might say, "It's nice to meet you, Kris" or "What are you up to, Kris?" I also visualize their name underneath their face, kind of like a picture with a caption below it. Again, I am a very visual learner. If I hear something, it is gone—but if I see it, I am good to go.

Knowing how I learn best has been instrumental in my success during my doctoral program. Prior to being diagnosed with ADHD, I always knew that I had trouble learning information that is presented auditorily; however, it wasn't until after my official assessment during my master's program that I realized that I was primarily a visual learner. Since that time, I have gotten into the habit of asking people to show me things, rather than explain them. For example, if somebody is giving me directions to get to a particular destination, I have them draw me a map. Even if they "draw" it in the air, it helps me more than had I just listened to them. Further, when studying, I have learned to use visual methods, such as flash cards and thematic mapping.

Of course, I couldn't have improved my ability to learn without self-reflection. Too often, people with ADHD are very passive about what is happening to them. They merely accept their present as being a prelude to their future. But that is not the case. We have the power to change, to adapt, to learn, to grow, to be better. Understanding oneself is the most important step on this lifelong journey.

I highly recommend that individuals with ADHD keep a journal and write every day. They should write about the things that help them learn and concentrate as well on what distracts them or prevents them from completing tasks. They should be allowed and encouraged to try new strategies, such as reading with the television or radio on. But they also have to be held accountable for their productivity, or lack thereof.

14

STRATEGIES FOR BUILDING EMOTIONAL SUPPORT

In the movie *Harvey*, Jimmy Stewart played a lovable drunk named El-wood P. Dowd. What is remarkable about Elwood is that his best friend is a giant white rabbit named Harvey who happens to be invisible. Throughout the movie, everybody thinks that he is crazy, so they want to institutionalize him and dope him up with drugs that will rid him of his "delusions." There is a scene where Jimmy Stewart faces everybody and says something like, "You know, I have been told that in order to get by in this life you need to be either really smart or really pleasant. Well, I have been really smart and, personally, I recommend being really pleasant." I am sure that isn't a direct quote, but it is the gist of what was said.

I love that scene and I use it regularly in my books and presentations. Whenever I think of it, I get goose bumps and have to smile. However, its full wisdom didn't hit me until a couple of summers ago.

Late one night during the summer of 2001, I went to the bathroom, looked down, and realized that I was peeing blood. Not just a little blood, but *a lot* of it. There was a large puddle of blood with red chunks floating in the toilet. The sight startled me, to say the least.

Immediately, I called "Ask a Nurse," which is a service where you can talk to a nurse on duty and get medical advice. I explained to her what had happened. Even though I was feeling perfectly fine, she instructed me to go to the emergency room right away.

After waiting several hours, I was finally able to speak with a doctor. He was very young and clearly tired, given that it was well after midnight. I explained what had happened and he looked somewhat concerned, especially when I told him that the urine wasn't just slightly reddish, but thick like catsup. He had me pee in a cup and ran some tests as I waited.

When he came back, he sat down on a stool in front of me. He no longer looked tired, but very worried. He said that there was a great deal of blood in my urine and that something was wrong. Of course, I already knew that and I wasn't even an M.D.!

He asked me how often I urinated. Ironically, this has always been a source of many jokes that my friends make at my expense. You see, I have a bladder the size of a thimble. I literally pee fifteen to twenty times a day if not more (apparently the average is six or seven). I pee so frequently that I rarely see a movie without taking at least one bathroom break! When I told the doctor this, he didn't look surprised or amused.

He then started asking about my family's medical history. When I reported that a couple of my grandparents had died of cancer, he began nodding gravely. He was particularly bothered by the fact that my maternal grandfather died at a relatively young age of prostate or bladder cancer, I couldn't remember which.

When I pressed him about what was wrong, he reluctantly said that I could have a tumor in my bladder and that he didn't like the sound of my family history. When I pushed harder, he said, "Yes, there is a slight chance of some sort of cancer." It would be rare in somebody my age, but given the history, the ongoing need to pee frequently, and the sheer volume of blood that I was expelling, he had a "bad feeling."

Being thirty-two years old and hearing the word "cancer" scared the crap out of me. When I told people, I put on a brave face and made jokes, but I was terrified. Things were just starting to look up for me. I had a job that I liked, a girlfriend whom I loved, and I was finishing my first book. Despite thinking about death for most of my life, I didn't want to die—not now.

Perhaps this sounds like a strange topic to be discussing, but it is immensely important. You see, people with ADHD, such as myself, suffer from high rates of depression. We abuse drugs and alcohol and attempt suicide more than the general population. As I have explained, ADHD affects more than just academic and social aspects of life. It can grind away at a child's self-esteem and make him or her feel like a loser or a failure. For this reason, it is crucial to help students with ADHD not only academically but emotionally as well. In fact, I would argue that the emotional development of children with ADHD is far more important than their academic development. After all, people can always learn to read or do math at any point in their lives. Changing their self-concept once in adulthood is much harder.

When I heard the doctor say "cancer," my attitude changed overnight. I wasn't going to let myself squander my life dwelling on negative emotions. I realized that time was too short and that I had to make a conscious effort to be happier.

In this chapter, I want to talk about what I have done over the past couple of years to address the emotional impact that ADHD has had on me. Please know that I still have problems with depression. I still "hear" my mother saying that I am a rotten kid. I hear echoes of my teachers saying that I need to try harder or apply myself. Many of my thoughts are negative and I find very little satisfaction in my successes.

Despite these difficulties, I have found the love of my life and I am happier now than I ever have been. I have to say that, like Elwood P. Dowd, I would rather be happy than smart. I have wasted so much of my life hiding in bathrooms and feeling miserable. When I left the emergency room two summers ago, I made a decision not to throw away any more time.

Clearly, one of the major factors for my transformation was having a doctor say "cancer." That was a real eye-opener. But it took more than a desire to be cheerful. I also developed strategies to help me maintain a positive attitude.

The first thing that I did was to sit down and think about what makes me happy. I actually made a list. Whenever I start feeling down, I do one of the things that I wrote down. For instance, I love animals. Perhaps what brings me the greatest joy in life is going to the Humane Society and walking some of the dogs. Some people say that seeing all of those homeless animals would be disheartening, but it isn't for me. They love the attention so much that they show it in their eyes. Further, no matter how bad things in my life get, seeing the animals without anybody to love them, without a place to call home except a small, filthy, concrete-and-wire kennel, I realize that my life is pretty damned good.

Another huge weapon that I have against depression is exercise. I try to work out every day. It doesn't take much, just fifteen to twenty minutes. Sometimes I lift weights, other times I walk on a treadmill. Not only does regular exercise make me feel better about myself, it helps me be able to sit down and concentrate far more than the medication that I have taken. Whenever I start feeling down about myself, I jump on a stationary bike for a few minutes and I feel better almost immediately.

In fact, exercise has worked so well for me, I started conducting research on whether it helps other people. Thus far, it seems very promising. I think my next academic endeavor is to see if exercise could be used to effectively treat ADHD instead of medication. Of course, I won't get any grants from the pharmaceutical companies!

Another factor contributing to my recent happiness involves self-reflection. In addition to actively thinking about what makes me happy and where I study best, I have been very good about reflecting on what is bothering me. As I have said before, my brain is like a wall full of televisions, each playing a different channel. Sometimes one of the television sets gets stuck on a very negative "show," such as my mother saying that I am a rotten kid or a past girlfriend calling me a loser. Sometimes the "show" isn't even based on reality. It is just playing a made-up thought that never really happened, or maybe it started playing an actual memory, but after spinning around my head for so long, it becomes distorted to such a degree that it no longer resembles what actually occurred.

This is an extremely important issue, so I need to explain it thoroughly. My thoughts are so real, so vivid, that they sometimes overwhelm me. I am often a slave to whatever image pops into my head. I could be fine one minute and then a sad or angry thought will begin circling in my mind. Almost instantaneously, I begin to feel that emotion wash over me.

For instance, and this probably sounds crazy, if I close my eyes and picture rain, I can feel it hitting my body. I literally can feel the imaginary water matting my hair and sliding down my back. I can feel the dampness, the chill, the impact. It is like I am really standing in the rain, the feeling is *that* powerful.

As you can imagine, having negative thoughts spinning out of control, whether real or not, has a profound impact on me. They make me feel down and depressed, even—when I was younger—suicidal. So I had to learn how to "change the channel." But that is not as easy as it sounds. People with ADHD tend to obsess on things. We have so many thoughts and we can't merely let go of them. They go round and round in our heads, getting more and more intense. As hard as we try, we can't push these thoughts out of our minds. In fact, the harder I tried to push them out, the more powerful they became.

Most of the counselors and therapists that I have seen didn't understand this. They seem to think that I could just "stop thinking." Several have even said that I shouldn't "think so much." First of all, I can't stop thinking. Second of all, I don't want to stop thinking, I just want to think of happier and more productive things. I want to change the channel, not get rid of the TV.

The first step in changing these bad channels is to realize that they are just thoughts. I frequently have to say to myself, "Rob, this isn't happening. You are sitting in front of your computer and what is going on in your head is just a memory (or it never happened at all)."

This is called "self-talk" and I use it a lot. Sometimes I even talk to myself out loud. It sounds nuts, but it works.

Another thing that I do to change bad channels is overcome them with good thoughts. This is different than trying to force the thoughts out of my head. As I said, I can't simply just stop thinking about the bad things. I can't just let them go. Once they are in my head, they are extremely difficult to dislodge. But I *can* replace them.

One of the quickest ways for me to change a bad channel into a good one is getting in my car, cranking the stereo as loud as it will go, and playing one of my favorite songs. The song that I play depends upon my mood. I am really partial to those that I can scream along to, such as "Twist and Shout." But softer, slower, more emotional songs such as "Imagine" and "In My Life" also do the trick. Christmas songs are effective all year round. Singing "White Christmas" along with Bing Crosby always makes me feel good.

In addition to singing in my car, I also like watching uplifting movies. Whenever I am depressed, I like watching the last fifteen minutes of *Rocky*. Rocky is getting knocked around. They have to cut his eye so he can see, but he is still standing and asking for more. The music starts building and he fights back. He is about to win when the bell rings and he discovers that he is a winner without having won the fight. How can anybody not feel good after watching that scene?!?!

It's a Wonderful Life is also one of my favorites. I can't imagine anybody feeling down after seeing George Bailey standing with his family and friends by the Christmas tree. Other movies that I watch regularly include *Mr. Holland's Opus*, *Backbeat*, *The Fisher King*, and *Tuesdays with Morrie*.

My friends also help me keep a positive mental attitude. I have never had many friends. I still only have a few. For a long time, this was a source of great disappointment for me. I always wanted to be popular and well liked. However, at some point I realized that, although I do not have a lot of friends, the ones that I do have have been by my side through some pretty tough times and I love them dearly for it. I try telling them that as much as possible.

As I think about my small group of friends, I find that they have several characteristics in common. First and foremost, they treat me very well. They might tease me or make fun of me for the strange things that I do, but they aren't mean. They never hit below the belt and they always seem to know when to back off and when to kick me in the butt. The Scholz girls are good examples. I have known them for my entire life, but I cannot remember one negative thing that they have ever said to me.

My friends are also pretty low key. They don't get extremely emotional one way or another. They really balance me out in that respect. When I get all sappy and emotional, they look at me and tell me to snap out of it. It sounds kind of harsh, but I know that they love me, too.

You may think that my good friends would understand me better than anybody else, but as I think about each one of them, they really don't. Only one or two of my close friends seems to know that I have ADHD. I might have told the others, but such things don't interest them. I have tried explaining why I do the things that I do, but they don't get it.

For a long time, I was really hurt by the fact that people, especially my friends and family, didn't understand. More than anything in the world, I have always wanted to be understood. But then I realized that being accepted is far more important and my friends do accept me for

STRATEGIES FOR BUILDING EMOTIONAL SUPPORT

who I am. Actually, the fact that my friends accept me even though they don't understand me makes them seem all the more special. When I do or say something stupid, they don't think "Oh, that is just the ADHD-thing talking." They think, "That is just Rob." It feels good to be around people who like me for who I am, not tolerate me despite my "disability."

My friends also tend to be fairly positive about life. This helps me a great deal. I can't stand being around negative people, even though I had been one for so many years. I am a firm believer that positive thoughts breed positive feelings.

Just as I try to value my small, close-knit group of friends, I try to stay away from people who are negative. Unfortunately, this isn't that easy because some of my family members and coworkers are perpetual worriers and breeders of negative thoughts. It is very hard for me to be around these people. I am like an emotional sponge—I pick up the negative vibes of those around me. So when I am talking to somebody who is unhappy with his or her life, I walk away feeling badly, too. Consequently, I try not to be around certain people for very long.

Journaling helps me a lot. Not only does it enable me to get things out of my head, but it also helps me determine which strategies work and which don't. For instance, as I look back on over fifteen years of journals, I see various themes emerge. I see what kinds of things bother me and what makes me happy. I realize that I have made some of the same mistakes in relationships and what kinds of people I should avoid in the future.

Perhaps the best thing about journals is that they are like emotional snapshots of my life. Sometimes I twist reality and I remember things far worse than they really were. Going back and reading what actually happened helps put things in perspective. It also helps me remember that, while I get depressed from time to time, those feelings always pass. "This will pass" is almost like a mantra for me when I am depressed. When I am in a depressed state, it feels like I have never been happy before. Reading my journal helps me realize that this isn't true.

Along the same lines of keeping a journal, I try to keep nice cards and e-mails that people send me. Whenever I start feeling like I am a loser, I pull some of them out of my drawer and read them. They really help. In fact, in front of me right now, taped to the top of my computer screen, is a note from my girlfriend, Daisey. All it says is, "You have a very good heart and you will accomplish everything you want in life." Every once in a while, I make myself read and really process it. I don't just read the words. I allow myself to feel the emotion behind it. I let the "goodness" of it sink in. You might say that I meditate on it. Doing so always makes me smile.

Improving myself is a journey. I had to let go of the idea that I will someday learn the "secret" that will make everything "perfect." Instead, I have gotten used to the idea of constantly looking for strategies and philosophies. I love listening to how other people see the world and deal with their problems. I also read a lot of biographies and self-help books. Sometimes they contain inspirational stories and useful strategies that I can use to improve my life.

Recently, I have become interested in a process called "creative visualization." It can be used for many things, but basically it involves imagining positive outcomes. For example, if I am nervous about teaching a class, I picture myself in front of the class with all of my students smiling and following along.

Creative visualization has really helped me when I get upset. If somebody yells at me or tells me that I am stupid, I don't let it affect me as much as it used to. I picture myself in a nice safe, comfortable place, such as a beautiful tropical island or the top of a snowy mountain. I then picture myself calmly talking to the person with whom I have the argument. It takes a lot of practice to internalize, but it seems to be helping me deal with stress.

I also use creative visualization to keep from getting bored. For example, if I am standing in line or trapped in a traffic jam, I tend to get frustrated very quickly. I can only stand around for a few minutes before I start getting angry. I hate waiting. It makes me feel like I am about to explode!! When I find that I have to wait, I like to daydream. I picture myself presenting to a large group of parents who are all cheering. Or I imagine that I am one of the Beatles. Most often, I pretend that I am a character in one of Tolkien's books. I can picture Middle Earth so clearly in my mind it is like I am there and I am no longer bored.

I use creative visualization to keep myself in a positive mind-set and to pull myself away from depression. The trick is not to focus on negatives. Sometimes this is difficult, especially when I want to rehash all the crappy events of my life rather than thinking about positive things.

Another area that I am working on lately is reveling in my successes. My failures last a lifetime, but my triumphs are gone within seconds. For instance, I have always dreamt about writing a book. I have been writing since elementary school. I first began submitting stories to publishers when I was in seventh grade. So you would think that seeing my first book on shelves in bookstores would generate some sense of joy, but it doesn't. I just think, "It could have been better" or "Let's see if it helps anybody."

I am trying to get out of that negative mind-set. I have been taking a few minutes out of every day to focus on all of the good things that I have done. I have to cringe about it sometimes. It makes me feel like I am bragging and I hate braggers. But I also have to take the time to enjoy my success, because nobody else can. They are *my* successes and life is meant to be enjoyed.

I want to end this chapter by reiterating the importance of building the self-esteem of children with ADHD. People can acquire academic skills at any point during their lives. If you are ninety years old and you want to learn about the Civil War, you can pick up a book, watch PBS, or take a class at your local college. Changing one's self-concept is far more difficult. Our conception of ourselves is basically fully formed once we leave elementary school. If you think that you are a loser when you are in seventh grade, chances are you will think that you are a loser when you are seventy. So please, if you are working with children with ADHD, address their academic needs, but don't forget about their emotional development. It is the best thing that you can do for them in the long run.

⓯

A LOOK BEHIND

Looking back, I am amazed by the twists and turns that my life has taken. It is remarkable to me that I have come so far and have seen so many different aspects of myself. For many years I thought that I was a loser and that I was slowly going crazy, but then I found out that I had ADHD. Eventually I was able to not only accept ADHD but also turn it into a valuable tool. The progression, however, was not a quick or easy one.

From the beginning, I was clearly different from my brothers. I was hyperactive even as an infant. Plus, once I started crawling, I was into everything. That is probably one thing that hasn't changed much; I am still very active. I have learned to sit and concentrate longer, but I can't just sit for the sake of sitting. I have to be constantly doing something productive. Boredom is hell for me and always has been. Most of the times that I got into trouble at school were when I was getting bored and looking for something to do.

When I first began attending school, I was actually excited and wanted to learn. In fact, I can still remember coming home from pre-school and informing my mother rather proudly that I was "the smartest boy in the class!" I used to ask a lot of questions about everything, not to be a pest, but because I really wanted to know. That enthusiasm

quickly left me, or was beaten out of me by the continual academic failure that was soon to follow. Of course, having teacher after teacher tell
me that I wasn't "living up to my potential" and that I should "try
harder" didn't help me either.

By fifth grade or so, I gave up academically. I was no longer the
smartest boy in class or anywhere else for that matter. I was no longer interested in learning. I stopped asking the persistent stream of questions
about everything under the sun. All that I wanted was to be left alone.

Quite frankly, I don't think that my teachers ever really cared if I
learned or not. They were more concerned about decreasing my disruptive behavior than fulfilling my intellectual potential. Further, by
eighth grade, my parents seem to have given up as well. As long as I
passed my classes, they didn't say anything. They were tired of the struggle as much as I was.

Initially, I was not only excited about school, but I was also a happy,
outgoing child. I was full of life and had a spirit that drove me to explore
everything around me. I also had a spirit that drove people crazy. In fact,
I giggled so much at the dinner table that my father spanked me.

During the first few years of elementary school, my teachers described me as socially immature. I talked when I wasn't supposed to. I
asked what they thought were silly, off-topic questions. I played the
same practical jokes over and over again until they lost any resemblance
of being funny. But I *was* social. I interacted. I laughed. I joked. I par-
ticipated in class.

By fourth grade or so, I began changing. Just as the continued academic failure extinguished my intellectual curiosity, the constant teasing
from my peers and frequent reprimands from my teachers and parents
for my behavior made me sullen and grim. I was becoming depressed
and isolated.

Eighth grade was a pivotal time for me. I was having a tremendous
amount of difficulties at school, both socially and academically. I had no
friends. I was extremely shy around girls and was barely passing my
classes. Plus, I had dropped out of church, causing a huge rift between
me and my family. The constant pain and anxiety of living had given way
to numbness. Before junior high had ended, I twice tried to kill myself.

By my sophomore year in college, I became more outgoing and more
confident. I began asking girls out and had a small group of friends. My

grades even improved and I was better able to focus the many thoughts that constantly swirled around in my head.

But this was just a fake Rob that was released whenever a bottle of schnapps or pitcher of beer had been emptied. I was still dark and moody, but as long as I had a few drinks in me, I didn't care what people thought. I could be rejected by a girl and then laugh about it at the bar.

Although alcohol masked my depression, it also unleashed potentially dangerous behavior. When drinking, I acted on all of my impulsive thoughts. I looked for fights and came close to hurting both friends and strangers. Though drinking helped me in many ways, it became obvious that its costs were eventually going to be too high for me to pay. I would probably have killed somebody if I had kept drinking. Plus, the depression was just covered over. It was still there and growing.

Despite the fact that research has clearly linked depression and ADHD, it was not the worst part of having ADHD. Depression ebbs and flows. It can be glossed over briefly by a strong drink, a brisk work-out, or a good cry. I have dealt with it throughout my entire life. Although I still feel myself slip into dark moods periodically, I am now a much happier person than I ever have been.

For me, the worst part of ADHD is not the depression but the effects that it has had on my self-esteem and self-concept. I am now in my mid-thirties. I have earned a Ph.D. from a good university. I have written five books and countless articles. I have presented all over the country. I have even written reports for congressional subcommittees. I have walked across the Pyrenees, fallen in love, bought my own home, and accomplished most of my dreams.

Despite my "successes," I still feel like a loser and that I can't do anything right. I still have self-deprecating thoughts in my head like a horde of vultures constantly circling on the edge of my mind. I still can't take much pleasure in what I do well because I remember all of my life's many failures. I still hear the echoes of all the people who have yelled at or made fun of me. "Jesus Christ, give me strength! You are such a rotten kid!" "If you just try harder you wouldn't get into so much trouble!" "You are so different!" Not a day goes by that I don't hear these at least once. I am in my thirties, but I sometimes still see myself as the little monster who terrorized his parents or the boy who hid in the bathroom when everybody else was playing during recess.

Poor self-esteem is very typical among people with ADHD. This is why we have such high rates of drug and alcohol abuse as well as suicide and divorce. Still, I do not believe that ADHD is solely to blame.

ADHD causes us to fixate on things. We constantly have multiple thoughts racing through our heads. Many times thoughts get stuck in our heads and they go round and round to the point of driving us mad. We also tend to have a great deal of energy that needs to be expelled. Because of this, we tend to have addictive personalities. We latch on to routines and rituals and perform them compulsively.

But it is not ADHD that makes our thoughts negative or our actions destructive. Most of the problems are caused by how people respond to us and our ADHD. My parents, teachers, and peers ridiculed and made fun of me. Their criticisms have been bouncing around my head ever since. Had they been more supportive or said, "Hey, you are all right. You are a good person," I would have learned to be happier a lot earlier on in my life.

Every month or so, I present at a conference or put on at least one workshop about ADHD. I particularly enjoy telling people what it was like growing up with ADHD. I tell my silly stories and explain some of the strategies that have helped me get to where I am. Sometimes people laugh. Sometimes they cry. After each presentation, I stand around and answer people's personal questions. Usually somebody will ask, "If you could go back and do it all again, would you do anything differently?"

This is a really good question, but it is difficult to answer. For one of the first times in my life, I like who I am. Things are going well for me and I am genuinely happy most of the time. Who I am now is largely due to who I was back then, so changing the past would change my present, which I don't want to do.

Still, as I look back on the little monster, I get somewhat sad, disappointed, and angry. As I prepared to write this book, I went through dozens of journals that I have kept throughout the years, read notes that my teachers sent to my parents, and rehashed things that I haven't thought about in many years. Some of these thoughts were good and made me laugh; many made me very disheartened and hurt.

When I examined my school records and notes from teachers, I have to wonder why they didn't help me more. Clearly I had problems. I wasn't mentally retarded, but I definitely had some difficulties learning and controlling my behavior. I realize that in the mid-1970s, special education was not what it is now. Kids only got special services if they had obvious disabilities, such as Down syndrome or cerebral palsy, but certainly they could have done more than simply putting me in the hallway or having me measure the school with a yardstick.

Of course, the next question is, "Should they have put you in special education?" And my honest answer is, "I don't know." That might sound a bit funny coming from a professor in special education. You probably would expect that I would rant and rave about how wonderful special education is, but I am not too sure.

Yes, special education can help a lot of students, especially if teachers take the time to figure out what is going wrong and what can be done to help the individual child. Unfortunately, it has been my experience that most special education programs only water down the regular curriculum and focus on remediation. This wouldn't have helped me. I wasn't a stupid kid. I didn't need things to go slower. In fact, I probably needed them to go faster. School bored me. I wanted more hands-on activities, more applied lessons. I wanted people to answer my many questions or to give me the skills to find my own solutions. Traditionally, special education doesn't do this.

Further, special education teachers tend to focus on compliance training. Rather than teaching students with ADHD how to utilize their energies in a productive way, they attempt to force them to sit still and pay attention. This is why so many special educators pressure parents into having their kids medicated.

Medication is another hot topic. I can't present anywhere without somebody asking me where I stand on it. Again, the answer is a bit convoluted.

I was on various medications for about ten years. Unfortunately, one of them caused me to have vocal tics which, even years later, haven't gone away. Much like somebody with Tourette's, I will sometimes blurt out words or sounds. For example, sometimes I will say "hello" like a startled parrot. Other times I bark like a dog. This is a common side effect of medications for ADHD, although many parents don't realize it.

Still, medications helped me in a number of ways. They increased my ability to pay attention. They also decreased, although only slightly, my hyperactivity. Perhaps most important, medications helped me keep my depression in check.

Nevertheless, I have to shake my head when I see what is going on in schools today. Kids line up in the office, waiting for their Ritalin. Meanwhile, nobody is teaching them how to change their behavior or trying to use other, nonmedicinal treatments, such as regular exercise or self-monitoring strategies.

I should point out that I am not a medical doctor. I have a Ph.D. in special education. Although I have researched medications for ADHD, M.D.s know a whole hell of a lot more than I do regarding pharmaceuticals. Regretfully, M.D.s do not seem to know much about ADHD. I have yet to meet a neurologist or a pediatrician who knew that ADD was no longer an accepted diagnosis from the American Psychological Association.

Further, M.D.s diagnose children with ADHD simply by taking the word of the parent or teacher. They do not observe children in multiple environments and over time. They don't conduct brain scans. They don't have the children take the computer-based tests that I had taken back in the 1990s.

Of course, this is to be expected. Medical professionals are overworked as it is. Nor can they be expected to be current on every single disability and illness. The same is true for special educators. Few educators seem to know about the changes in diagnostic criteria for ADHD.

When it comes to medication, I have to defer to the medical doctors. Hopefully they have taken it on themselves to be current and to at least ask some basic questions, such as "What behavior modification strategies have you tried?" before prescribing anything.

When talking to parents and teachers, I recommend that they find doctors who do not prescribe medications without first trying other strategies. Further, if a doctor talks about "ADD," parents should probably look elsewhere for medical advice. As we mentioned in one of the first chapters, ADD stopped being used as a legitimate diagnosis nearly a decade ago. If they mention it, their knowledge is clearly not up to date.

I also do not recommend that young children be put on medications. Again, I am not a medical doctor and every situation is different. Still, with the growing evidence that drugs for ADHD can have severe and irreversible side effects, I do not feel comfortable with four- and five-year-olds taking medication—but that is just me. Other professionals with just as much experience have other points of view.

In fact, the debates about medication can become very vocal and personal. During an interview that I gave to a reporter, I mentioned that I thought medication should be used as a last resort. Soon after the article was published, a physician called and started yelling at me. "Who the hell do you think you are doling out medical advice?!?! Are you a doctor?"

The physician and I talked for about half an hour. I tried explaining to him that, while I was not a medical doctor, I was aware of many studies that found that various medications for ADHD had very serious side effects and that there are other methods of helping children concentrate and be productive than drugs. He countered that medication is safe in an overwhelming majority of the cases and that by delaying medication children just fall further and further behind in school.

His point is a valid one. The long-term risks of medication are rare; however, they are not rare enough if your child is the one out of a hundred who develops brain damage or liver failure or dies. Further, I feel that medication should only be used in conjunction with other strategies, such as behavior modification. Moreover, medication should be used when all else fails. In the end, parents have to weigh the risks with the potential benefits. It is their decision whether or not to medicate their child, not the decision of Ph.D.s, M.D.s, teachers, or the media.

As I look back over the past thirty-something years, I learn a lot about myself and my social life. It has always been very hard for me to develop good and lasting friendships. Part of this is due to my insecurities. Whether it is because of my ADHD or just my personality, I am not very good with people I do not know. I never have a clue what to say when I meet people and I can't fake interest in what they tell me. I also usually say exactly what is on my mind, which is not a valued characteristic in our society.

Perhaps the most significant reason why I haven't had many good friends is that certain people are not very good for me. I tend to feed off other peoples' emotions. If somebody around me is happy and positive, I will feel happy and positive. But if he or she is negative or depressed, I will feel negative or depressed. As a result, I actively try to stay away from certain "types" of people, especially worriers or complainers.

In retrospect, I have lost a lot of friends after arguments over little things that became much bigger than they should have. I am incredibly sensitive. But I also don't fight fair. When I get into a minor tiff with somebody, I will say mean and hurtful things. I will say whatever comes to mind without regard to how the person will feel or how it will affect our future relationship.

Over the past couple of years, I have been working on my temper. Lately, it hasn't been a problem. Still, I am very likely to burn bridges and I struggle to keep things in perspective.

When I present at conferences, people also ask me about my family. Specifically, they ask how I get along with them now and what I would change about how I was raised. I hesitate to write about this, but I think that it is a very important topic to consider. Many people with ADHD whom I have met have explained that their relationships with their families haven't turned out well. I am afraid that this is very predictable.

My relationship with my family is difficult to describe. Given that I come from a pretty large family, at least for nowadays, I have to tell people that my relationship depends upon the specific family member. In general, my family isn't extremely close. Each of my brothers has moved to a different part of the country and three out of the five of us have wives and kids. Basically, we all have our own lives and don't interact much. We all get together whenever there is an important event, such as a wedding or a funeral. But, by and large, we only get all together every few years and we usually converse through our mother who relays what is happening through the Jergen grapevine.

In regard to my parents, I think that we have a better relationship now than when I was younger. I don't think that they are frustrated by my behavior anymore. They have gotten used to my many and changing interests as well as my impulsive need to relocate every year or two. When I talk about going on for another Ph.D., they just nod their heads and smile blandly.

I should point out that my parents and brothers don't mention much about my past. Once in a while somebody would say, "We were really concerned about you" or "You were such a handful." But that is about it. Actually, I prefer it this way. For the most part, thinking about how stupid I was makes me feel uncomfortable.

I should also point out that, to this day, my mother denies that I have ADHD. She says that I simply had problems sitting still, paying attention, doing things without thinking, and completing tasks once I started them. My brothers are pretty skeptical, as well. One of them told me that I act the way I do because I choose to and not because I have a "disability."

I guess that if I could change anything about my childhood or my relationship with my family, it would be how they supported me. My family is just like any other family. We love each other in our own unique ways. Unfortunately, we tend to show our love by picking on each other. Being the youngest and a bit odd to begin with, I tended to get the brunt of the teasing. This didn't help my self-esteem.

I wish they were more supportive of me even now. For instance, when I recently told two of my brothers that I suffer from depression and that I tried to kill myself in junior high, they didn't believe me. One of them said that I had no business thinking that my pain was any worse than anybody else's. The other said that I was "just trying to get attention." As a result, I try to stay away from any topics that are important to me, such as ADHD, politics, or philosophy. As far as they are concerned, I am Robbie, the melodramatic, hypersensitive freak. I don't think that they will ever see me as a successful doctor, author, or professor. They tend to minimize my successes rather than letting me savor them. For example, when I got a publishing contract for my first book, my mother said, "Well, let's see if you actually finish writing it." I think that I would have better self-esteem now if they had encouraged me more when I was growing up.

It is interesting to note that one of my nephews has been diagnosed with ADHD and none of my family members seems to question it. Actually, he has been diagnosed with ADD, which bothers me no end. I am not sure if he has ADHD. I haven't been around him much to develop an informed opinion. Moreover, his parents don't seem to want my perspective or expertise on the matter, so I don't bring it up.

One of the things that I would do differently is that I would try much harder in school. I admit that I gave up. That is my fault and nobody else's. If I just had applied myself, I think that I would be much more knowledgeable than I am today.

Further, I am not sure if I would have gone into special education. Don't get me wrong; I love what I do. I love teaching and writing. But I wish that I had gone into a more challenging field. Perhaps something involving science or mathematics, something that would have made a bigger impact on the world. I think that I would have been a good engineer or scientist. Maybe I could have looked into curing cancer or cleaning up pollution.

Also looking back, I also think that I should have been more selective when accepting jobs. Southwestern Missouri State University and the Institute on Developmental Disabilities didn't match my needs or interests. Still, I learned a lot from being there, which has helped me become happy where I am today.

When I look back, I wish that I wouldn't have ended some of the friendships that I once had. Most of the friendships that I have lost have been my fault. I said or did things that prevented any kind of reconciliation. Knowing this, however, has helped me maintain the few friendships that I have. I constantly try to tell my friends how much I love them and I value them beyond all else.

I would have also been more careful about the doctors and therapists that I went to. Some of them were horrible. For instance, a couple of therapists tried convincing me that I was abused as a child and that I had repressed all of the memories of it. This is not the case. My parents and brothers never touched me in any inappropriate way.

Moreover, it seems like every time I get a new doctor, he or she wants to diagnose me with something other than ADHD, such as bipolar personality disorder. They have even told me that my "success in school" (i.e., the fact that I earned a Ph.D.) "precludes me from having ADHD." Ugh!

However, the worst doctors were the ones who didn't answer my questions regarding the medications that they were prescribing. Some refused to answer my questions for whatever reasons. Others just didn't have the skill to explain things so that a layperson could understand them. As a result, I have had to take it upon myself to learn what I could through other means, such as the Internet and medical journals.

I think the bottom line is that, yes, parts of my past really sucked. I have experienced some pretty challenging and trying times. But who I am is largely ue to what my past was like and how I dealt with it. Further, my present is pretty damned good and my future will be even better—if I continue to learn from my past.

A LOOK FORWARD

When I think about my future, I am far more optimistic than I ever have been before. In and of itself, that is a magnificent thing! I spent far too much of my life worrying and feeling bad about myself. I have frittered away too much time struggling socially, academically, and professionally.

As with the past and the present, I realize that there are going to be times when the future won't be so great. I know that I will experience periods of depression and that my ADHD will cause me to do or say something stupid. I know that there will be times when I will sit in front of my computer and not be able to form a coherent sentence. I know that there will always be people who don't understand me or who even hate my guts because of my behavior. All of this, I know.

I also know that much of my life is under my control and not anybody else's. I know that there are ways of making ADHD a good thing. I just have to look for them. I know that I will meet people who are similar to me and that I am not alone. I know that things always work out for the best, if I am willing to make the best happen. Most important, I know that I am a good person and that I only need to keep trying in order to be better.

Right now, life is pretty good for me. Yes, the past has been full of anguish—the failures, the social isolation, the drinking, the suicide attempts. So, too, are portions of the present, as well as the future. But overall, I am content. The little monster is gone—at least for now. He visits my mind once in a while. Sometimes we sit and cry together. But at this very moment, life is wonderful.

I have to confess that there are some aspects of my future that concern me a little, such as interpersonal relationships. Although I am currently dating Daisey, sometimes it is a lot of work for her to be around me. We break up every six to eight weeks, most of the time because of something that I said or did, or didn't say or didn't do. For instance, Daisey was applying to be a foster parent. She asked me several times if I would write her a letter of recommendation, which I was more than happy to do. When she gave me the form, she said, "Don't lose it." I knew how important the form was to her. Despite my efforts, I lost it within two days. She was crushed. She thought that I did it on purpose or that I simply didn't care enough about her to keep track of a piece of paper.

Daisey knows about my ADHD. She has read my books and goes to great lengths to understand me. Yet, understanding the cause of the behavior doesn't take away what happens. It is much like somebody getting run over by a car. It doesn't matter why it happened; the person is still dead. And, unfortunately, I have a tendency to run over people's feelings without realizing it.

Another adult with ADHD told me a great story that illustrates this very well. Apparently he and his wife were at a county fair. It was a hot day and, being a very sweet guy, he asked his wife if she wanted something to drink. She said that she wanted some lemonade. So the husband, smiling and whistling, waits in line to get her a nice tall glass of tasty lemonade. By the time he gets to the front of the line, however, he forgets her drink and gets himself a beer. He then returns to the table where his wife is sitting. Seeing that, once again, her husband had forgotten about her, she gets mad. But the husband, being oblivious to his wife's subtle clues (e.g., arms folded, eyes flashing, teeth clenching), goes on drinking his beer as if nothing is wrong, which gets the wife even angrier.

The husband is an extremely kind and loving man. His wife is the first to say this. Further, she is a school counselor and works with kids with ADHD. She knows all about ADHD. She sees it every day at school. She understands why her husband does the things that he does. She understands that much of what he does is beyond his control. Still, she feels neglected and forgotten. Every day something like the lemonade incident happens in their relationship. Despite the cause, she can't take much more of it. She is thinking about divorcing him.

The point is, yes, ADHD might cause certain behaviors. And, yes, people might understand why these behaviors are occurring. But that realization and understanding doesn't take away the fact that the behaviors bother people. I am who I am and I try very hard to be a good person, but I still have to be aware that I annoy the crap out of people, especially the people I date, and my friends, family, and coworkers.

I guess that is why I can't imagine ever getting married. This is a recent revelation. Up until a couple years ago, I always thought that I would meet somebody, fall in love, get married, and have the perfect life—family meetings, bringing flowers home for no reason, telling my wife that I love her every single day. But lately, I have realized how insane I drive people. As much as I love them, as much as I try to be a good person, I can't envision being with somebody day in, day out for the rest of my life. It isn't that I don't want to share my life with somebody. It is just that I think that if I really loved somebody, I wouldn't subject her to my erratic behavior and oddities. It is kind of like the old W.C. Fields line, "I wouldn't be in a club that would have me as a member." I try to be a good boyfriend, but I know that Daisey needs a lot of time away from me. I can be a bit overwhelming, to say the least.

This isn't good or bad. It is simply how things are. People with ADHD have very high divorce rates, much higher than the national average. I don't want to get divorced or frustrate my loved ones. But more important, I have realized that I don't have to get married to be happy.

My view on kids has also changed recently. I have always wanted children. I even considered adopting a child on my own since I didn't think I would ever get married. I thought that I would be a good father. After all, I have a lot of energy and I am very emotional. Given my past, I think that I would be very supportive and nurturing. All of this is true. Yet, I just don't have the patience or the attention span to be a good parent.

I have trouble being around kids. Sure, they are fun for a little while—that is, when they aren't screaming or making noise for the sake of making noise! But you have to watch them all the time, especially when they are tiny. It is hard enough for me to pay attention to a half-hour television program, let alone a little kid. Further, I can't hide my emotions. While being emotional and caring is one of my strengths, I have a very low frustration level. I don't tolerate things very well. I can see myself getting angry, clenching my fists, looking up at the ceiling, and saying, "Jesus Christ, give me strength! You are such a rotten kid." I don't want to do that to anybody.

My employment future is constantly in doubt. I love being a professor. I love teaching and writing and working with my students. Even if I won the lottery, I would still be doing what I am doing. I don't think that I will ever retire. I will be one of those eighty-year-old professors who still thinks that he is twenty-five. In fact, nothing would please me more that to kick the bucket in class right in front of my students! It would certainly make an impact on them.

Still, I get bored very easily and special education doesn't hold my attention for long. After all, it isn't rocket science. There hasn't been a new thought of any significance in special education in decades. We are still arguing over the same questions, "What is intelligence?" "Can intelligence be measured?" "Should children with disabilities be taught alongside their nondisabled peers?" "What is the purpose of education?" Et cetera, et cetera, et cetera. As a field, we have the same debates over and over again and they bore me.

I am constantly thinking about going back to school and getting another Ph.D. I have looked into becoming a counselor or psychiatrist, but it was brought to my attention that I am not very good with people and can't listen for long, so maybe those aren't the fields for me. I actually started a second Ph.D. in economics when I was living in Chicago, but I moved away before I got very far into the program.

That is another problem that I have: I get very bored with my surroundings. Prior to my present position, I had not stayed at a job longer than a year. I get very restless and a strong compulsion to relocate grabs hold of me. The only reason I have been at the University of Wisconsin for more than a year is because I bought a house so I can't just pick up and move as easily as I used to.

Most adults with ADHD have the same problem. We find something new, get really excited about it, and then suddenly something else grabs our fancy so we forget about the first thing. Some adults with ADHD whom I know have quit their jobs on an impulse. They get an idea stuck in their head that they want to do such and such, so they see their boss walking down the hallway and say, "I quit!" They don't think about what they are saying or the ramifications of their actions.

I am not that bad, but I do look at the job postings every day. Every year, I have interviewed for a new job at one place or another. Fortunately, I have really bad interview skills and rarely get offered other positions. So, I am stuck here for good or for ill.

The fact that I know that I get antsy and will want to move has helped me. I know that this feeling will pass as soon as I find something else to dominate my attention. I also know that, in the future, I will want to pick up and move on the spur of the moment. To stop me from acting on every little whim, I don't keep copies of my vita. Every time I see a job and think, "I want to go there!" I have to retype my vita from scratch. This takes several days and prevents me from sending out applications every time the mood hits me. I also hate rewriting my vita and cover letters, so the thought of applying for jobs has become less palatable.

Since cultivating the belief that ADHD is a good thing, I have become very goal- and process-oriented. I constantly set objectives and then plan ways of achieving them. Without constantly having tasks to work on, I get stir crazy. I get bored and being bored is hell for me. Most of the trouble that I got into as a kid was when I was bored and didn't have anything to do. Further, focusing upon the process, rather than merely the outcome, forces me to pay attention to the details that I typically ignore or forget.

One of my goals is to start spreading my belief that ADHD is an asset and should be utilized rather than repressed. This has been one of my preoccupations over the past year. In addition to writing books, I have been presenting at various conferences and conducting workshops for parents and teachers. I am hoping that I can inspire at least a few people or help some kid with ADHD not make the same mistakes that I have made.

Although I currently feel that promoting ADHD as a good thing is very important, I also know that it will not hold my attention for very long. After I complete this book, I may never write about ADHD again. But then again, what do I know? My interests change like the wind. While some people say I can't stick to anything, I say that I want to explore the world!

I suppose that my principal goal is to be happy and to let the past be my past, not my present. Some days this is hard to do. I sometimes wallow in self-pity. I complain about how people treat me or have treated me in the distant past. I get frustrated because I can't do all the things that I want to do at the time when I want to do them. Having ADHD in a non-ADHD world is like walking through waist-deep water. You have to be patient. But I am not a patient person. I have learned that if I focus on enjoying the water, it makes the wading a little bit easier.

I hope that this book and the stories about my life have helped you in some way. If there is anything that I can leave you thinking about, it is that ADHD is a great condition to have. Yes, it has some bad points, but overall ADHD is a wonderful gift—if it is utilized!

17

SOME SUGGESTIONS FOR PARENTS, TEACHERS, AND PEOPLE WITH ADHD

After completing the first sixteen chapters of this book, I thought that I was more or less finished. I gave the drafts of what I had written to several of my students and friends. I wanted their sincere feedback about its writing style and content.

Daisey read a couple pages and then refused to go any farther. She said that it was "too painful" to read about my childhood and that hearing about it made her "extremely sad." My students, on the other hand, gave me glowing reviews. Some of them seemed genuine, but opinions of others were probably influenced by the fact that I was their professor. Perhaps they were afraid that I would lower their grade if they said something negative!

Somehow, my manuscript got into the hands of a parent. She called me up and, through what sounded like choking tears, explained her situation. She told me that her son was in fifth grade and that my book described him perfectly. As patiently as I could, I listened as she told me about how her son was diagnosed with ADHD "even though he is a good kid and very smart." She also explained that he was having problems in school. His grades were dropping and he no longer had any friends. What troubled her most was that she felt that he was "changing." She felt that he was becoming withdrawn and rarely came out of his room. She spoke to his teachers about it, but they said that he was just entering adolescence. After reading what I had written, she wasn't sure. She was afraid that he might be depressed and that he might try killing himself just as I had done when I was about his age. She concluded by begging me to tell her what to do.

Although I thought of several suggestions that I could have offered the woman, I was reluctant to mention them. I am always a bit hesitant to dispense advice. After all, who the hell am I to tell a parent what to do? She and her son clearly needed help. But I didn't know them and advice is often a dangerous gift to give. What if I was wrong and something bad happened? It would be my fault and I couldn't live with that, so I only gave her very general information.

I began by telling her about various organizations and support groups like CHADD and that she should have her child evaluated for depression by a trained professional. But she wanted something more specific that she could do to help her child. She kept pushing and pushing.

As I politely explained that I was willing to point her in a few directions, but that I didn't think that it was appropriate for me to tell her what to do, I heard a little voice in my head. It said, "I wish somebody would have helped me." It was my own voice. More precisely, it was the voice of the little monster.

Because of my conversation with the woman and the contact that I have had with her and her son since, I decided to add one more chapter to this book. Specifically, I want to discuss how I think parents and teachers can help children with ADHD. I also want to talk about how children with ADHD can help themselves.

I would like to stress in the strongest way possible that my suggestions will not work for everybody. In fact, they may not work for anybody but myself. Every situation is different. Just as medication is not a silver bullet that cures ADHD, nothing that I can say will make everything all right for everybody. Still, maybe I can be of some assistance in very broad terms.

ADHD has to be treated using a multiple-pronged approach. As I have stressed before, research has found that medication by itself is not very effective in helping people with ADHD. Other strategies need to be employed at the same time. After all, medications don't teach. They may help some people concentrate or sit still, but they will not show a child how to read or make him or her treat others with respect.

In my particular case, I took several different types of medications before I found something that worked for me. But I also developed ways of changing my environment so that I could be more productive. Further, I built support networks that helped me address the psychological aspects of having ADHD, especially the feelings of worthlessness and depression. Finally, I actively sought out and developed strategies that helped me learn. These approaches are discussed in detail within this book, so I will not revisit them. Still, there are some important things that I feel inclined to address in order to help the other little monsters who are out there.

First and foremost, I firmly believe that building a child's self-esteem is far more important than improving his academic abilities. This is simply my opinion. I have no empirical evidence to back this up or to prove my point beyond a shadow of a doubt. Further, other more educated people might disagree vehemently with me. Regardless, I believe that building the self-esteem of children is the most critical charge that parents and teachers have, especially when they are working with children who are at risk of depression and suicide.

As I have said several times before in this book, I can learn to read or do math at any point in my life. In fact, I just bought a computer program that is teaching me how to do algebra. I am also listening to a book on tape about ancient Rome. Eventually, I might take a class on how to speak Norwegian or how to play the guitar. Learning is not limited to schools or to childhood. It is a lifelong process. Additionally, I will forget how to spell words or how to divide fractions, but my self-esteem affects me each and every day.

Though people can learn throughout their entire lives, it is very difficult for them to change their self-concept once they become adults. It seems that once people leave junior high or high school, their personalities are pretty much set in stone. The stone can be chiseled, polished, or reshaped slightly, but you are limited in what you can make of it.

I have tried to change my self-concept and, to some degree, I have made significant progress. But, at times, I am still consumed by doubts and feelings of worthlessness. I no longer seriously consider killing myself; however, I don't see myself as "successful." Nor do I take great satisfaction in my accomplishments. Moreover, I don't try as many things as I would like simply because I think that I am going to fail at them. In fact, I think that I am hampered more by how I view myself than by my actual behavior or abilities.

If you are a parent or a teacher, my advice is to focus primarily on your child's self-esteem. I am not saying to abandon academics completely. I just want to emphasize the fact that knowledge is secondary to happiness; at least, it is in my mind. Think about it this way: Would you rather have a very smart but miserable child who is at risk of committing suicide, or a happy, well-adjusted child who is behind academically?

The question becomes, "How can parents and teachers build a child's self-esteem?" There are tons of books on the subject, and I am no expert, but it seems that the first thing is to be extra supportive. Be patient. And focus on the positive far more than the negative.

I know that we ADHDers bother normal people and make them want to pull their hair out, but I think that, for the most part, kids with ADHD try to be good. We want to be accepted and loved, just like everybody else. We try to avoid the punishments and ridicule. We just mess up more frequently than do our peers. If you focus on the positive, on the fact that we really are trying, our behavior becomes far more tolerable.

Further, keep in mind that every little negative comment that you let slip echoes in our heads for a very long time. We forget our schoolwork. We forget people's names. We forget to take the trash out. But we don't forget all of the crap people give us. Eventually, it sinks into our heads and it is nearly impossible to get it out. If you tell us that we are stupid or rotten, we will eventually become stupid or rotten.

Take time every day to tell your children all of the good things that they have accomplished. Make a list of their positive qualities and put it on the refrigerator door. Review and revise it often. Talk about all of the things that they can do and paint positive pictures of their futures.

Make accommodations for ADHD. Don't expect a child with ADHD to be able to sit still for hours on end. Don't give her boring tasks that require a lot of mental effort. Try utilizing different teaching strategies. Write directions down and post his responsibilities somewhere where he can see it. Get her into the habit of using her energies in productive ways. Allow frequent breaks. Overlook harmless comments and behaviors; they are meaningless compared to the big picture.

Although children with ADHD may need certain accommodations, they should *not* be allowed to use ADHD as an excuse for inappropriate behavior! They still must try in school, do their homework, and treat others with respect. Of course, getting kids to be nice is no easy feat even when they don't have ADHD. So how can teachers and parents produce happy children who are also good people?

As with anybody, children with ADHD must be taught what is expected of them and how to behave. This requires consistency and frequent reminders. I would recommend that you get a book on behavior modification, such as *Enhancing Your Child's Behavior: A Step-by-Step Behavior Modification Guide for Parents and Teachers*. This book will help you develop a systematic method for promoting the behaviors that you want and reducing the behaviors that you don't.

In addition to being consistent, parents and teachers must also expect and demand performance. This doesn't mean that children with ADHD have to do the same thing as their nondisabled peers. They may require modifications as a result of their inability to concentrate or sit still. Yet, a student with ADHD who is in third grade should be expected to do third grade work or better. Remember, ADHD doesn't mean "stupid." Individuals with ADHD are likely to be gifted, though their schoolwork may not show it.

Too often, parents and teachers focus on the amount of work that children are supposed to do, rather than whether a child has learned what is being taught. For example, imagine that a child with ADHD is assigned fifty math problems to complete over the weekend. If the child remembers to do it at all, he is likely to make a lot of careless mistakes, especially toward the end of the assignment. As a result, the child will probably do pretty poorly. Teachers and parents then interpret this to mean that the child can't do math. After all, he failed the assignment.

Rather than focusing upon the completion of assignments, teachers and parents should focus on acquisition of knowledge. For example, instead of giving a student fifty math problems, have her do ten. If the student can do all ten perfectly, then she is done. You can tell that she knows how to do math. But if she misses any, have her do another set of ten problems until she gets them all correct. Again, the emphasis is on assessing learning, not completion of work. Plus, from my experience, it seems that students find this approach highly motivating.

I also recommend that students be allowed to choose how they will demonstrate whether they have mastered a task. This means, if they don't do very well on paper-and-pencil tests, they can elect to present information orally. They can choose whatever way they want, but they must prove to teachers and parents that they know the content or have mastered the skill in question.

In addition to demanding and expecting appropriate behavior and academic performance, I also think that children should be told what ADHD is. Too often I have gone to schools and found that kids think that ADHD is another way of saying "mentally retarded." Moreover, it seems that a lot of kids say things like "I can't do that. I have ADHD" or "My ADHD made me do that."

When explaining what ADHD is, I think it is very important to focus on the positive. I don't mention the word "disability." I emphasize "difference." I also talk a lot about how ADHD is a good thing.

For example, when I am working with young children with ADHD, I begin by talking about superheroes or Pokémon. We chit-chat about various superheroes and how each of them has a different super ability. Superman can fly and is really strong. Batman has his gadgets. Spiderman can crawl up walks and shoot webs. And so on.

I then point out that people are just like superheroes. We all have our strengths and weaknesses. Some kids are really good at spelling. Others are good at kickball. Still others are funny or artistic.

People with ADHD are just like superheroes. They tend to be really smart. Plus, they have tons of energy and are creative. The trick is teaching them how to use their super abilities in positive and productive ways, much like Superman had to learn how to fly in order to save Lois Lane all the time. If kids with ADHD are not taught how to utilize their natural abilities, they end up bouncing off walls and being destructive, just like an undisciplined Clark Kent.

If you are an individual who is lucky enough to have ADHD, I say this: Don't expect other people to understand you. They won't. We are completely foreign to non-ADHDers and probably always will be.

Instead of understanding, look for love and admiration. Surround yourself with people who care for you because of who you are, not in spite of your diagnosis. These people will be few and far between, so do everything that you can to keep and maintain their friendships.

Also, do not expect other people to make your life better. You have to do it yourself. You have to find ways to make your life a success. You have to develop strategies that help you learn and function in a non-ADHD world. It is all up to you. Non-ADHD people, whether they are teachers, parents, or counselors, can't do it for you.

Moreover, find out about the medications that you are taking. Watch for side effects and ask your doctors questions. If you don't understand their answers, ask more questions, get another doctor, or look on the Internet. Medications can be very helpful, but they shouldn't be taken lightly. They can cause serious and permanent damage to your body. They can even kill you.

I also suggest that you join support groups, such as CHADD or ADDA (go to www.chadd.org and www.adda.org for more information). There are local chapters throughout the country. They also have annual state and national conferences that provide very useful information.

Support groups and professional organizations are also very beneficial because they enable you to talk with other people who have ADHD. Through them, you can see what helps other people. You can also see that you are not alone.

Additionally, I recommend that you experiment with your environment and learning strategies. See what works for you and what doesn't. Keep a journal and write in it regularly. Then go back and see how things have changed in your life and figure out why. The answers are out there. You just have to find them.

There is one last thing that I think everybody who is touched by ADHD needs to understand. In and of itself, ADHD is not bad. Yes, there are some downsides. We tend to have poor self-esteem, abuse drugs, and kill ourselves. But, overall, I personally believe it is a gift. It is a great source of energy and creativity. It makes life interesting and entertaining.

Whether you are a parent, teacher, counselor, social worker, pediatrician, or a person with ADHD, focus on reducing the negative aspects of ADHD and maximizing its potential benefits. Pick your battles and don't try to eliminate ADHD itself. Forcing a child to sit still, whether by medications or by punishment, does nothing to actually help the child. And above all, focus on being happy, not on trying to be "normal."

Good luck and thank you for reading this book. I hope it helped.